Alginates - Recent Uses of This Natural Polymer

Edited by Leonel Pereira

Published in London, United Kingdom

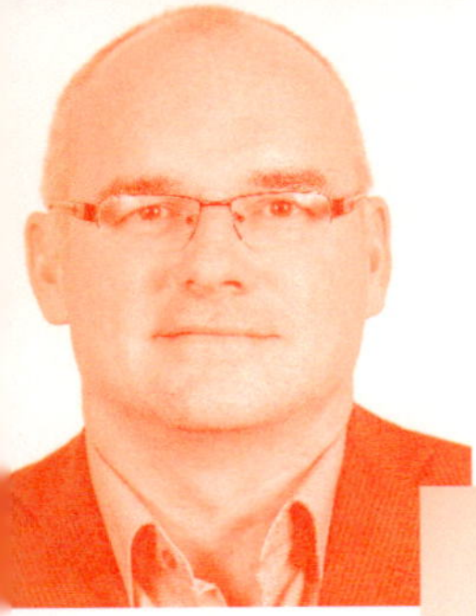
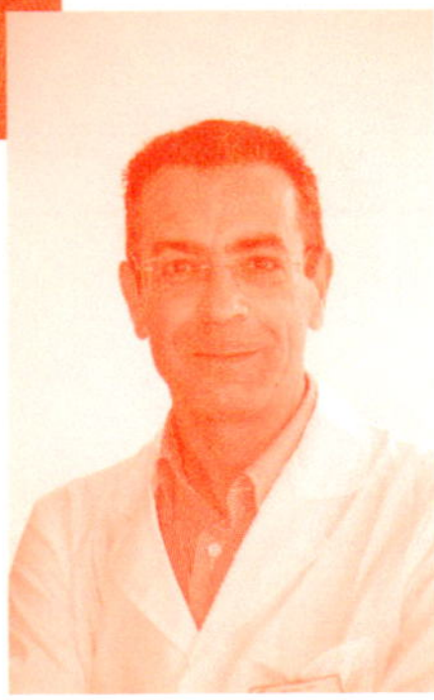
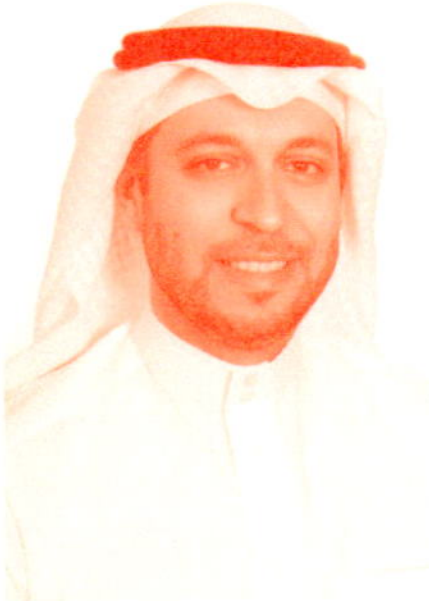
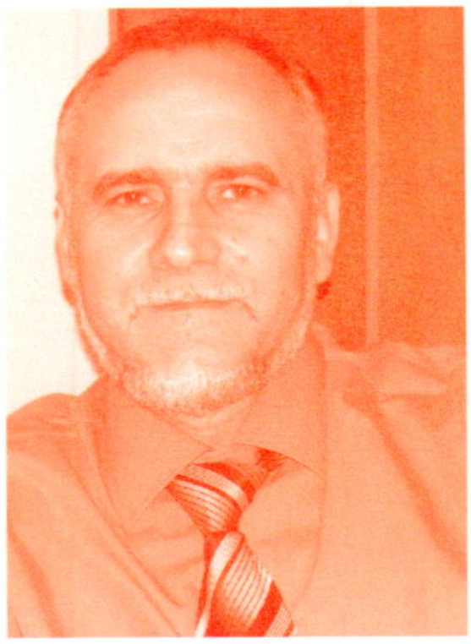
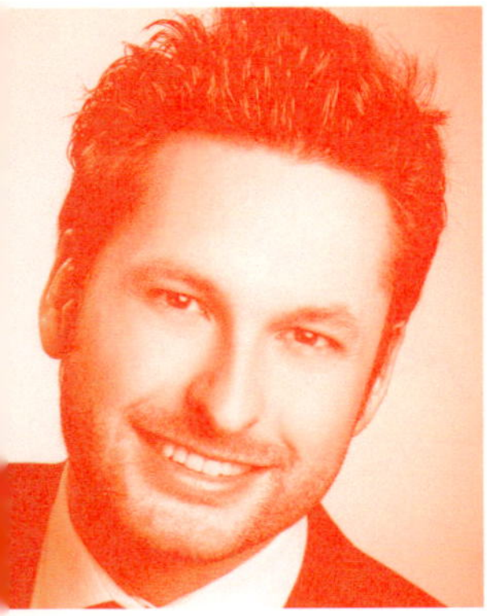
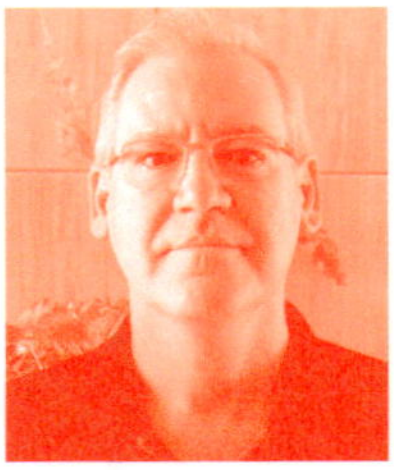
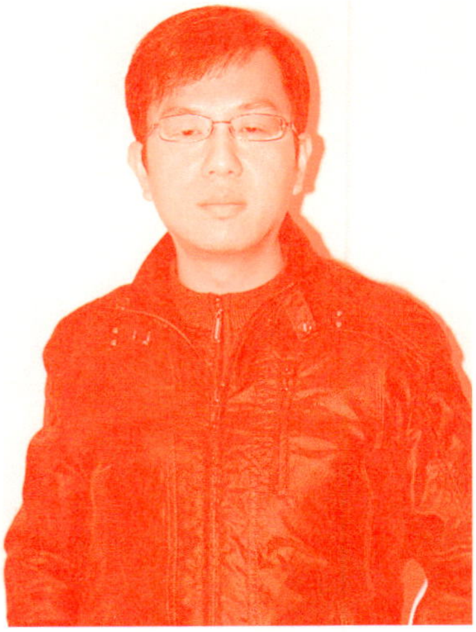

IntechOpen

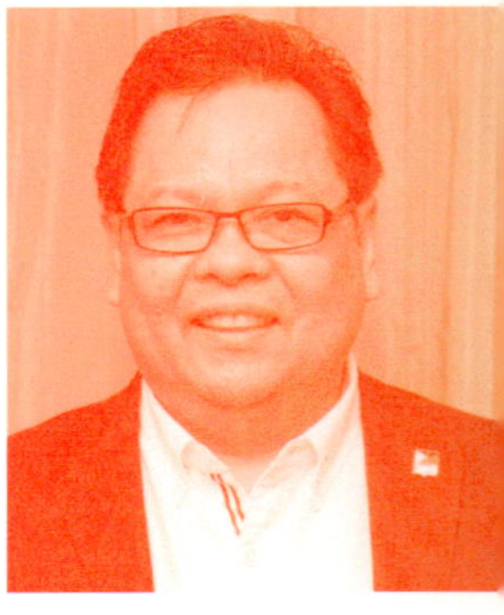
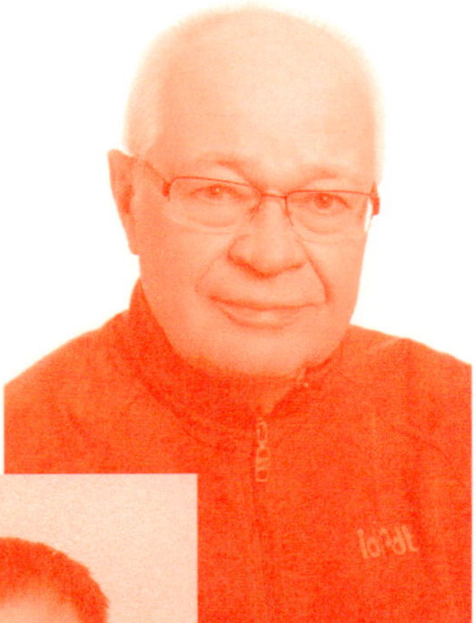
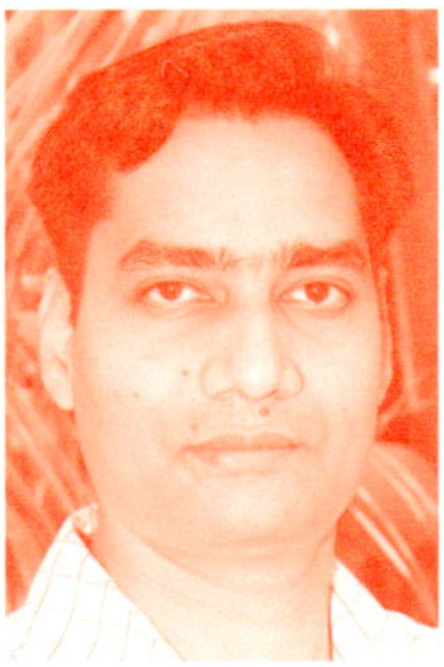
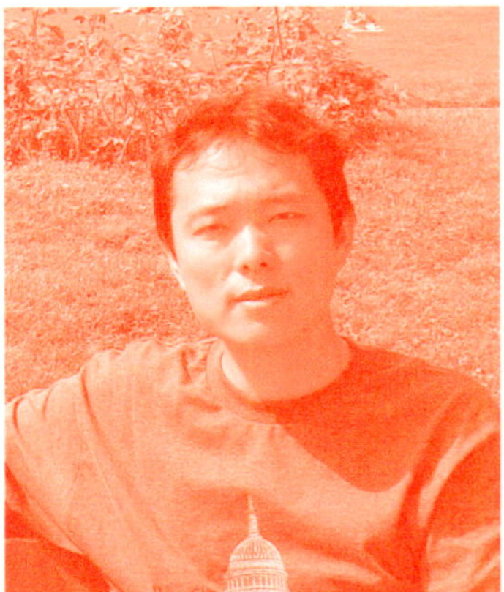
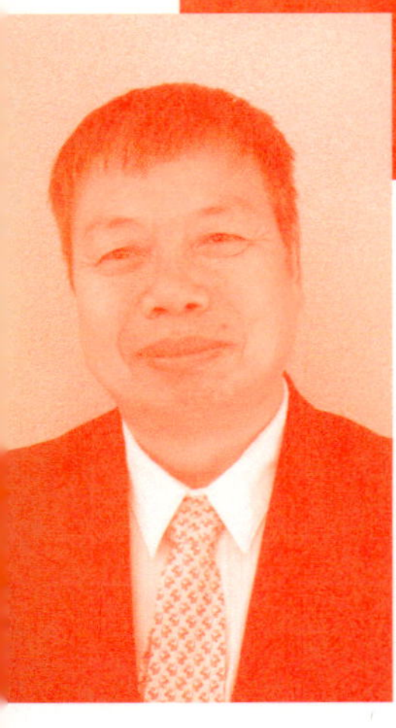
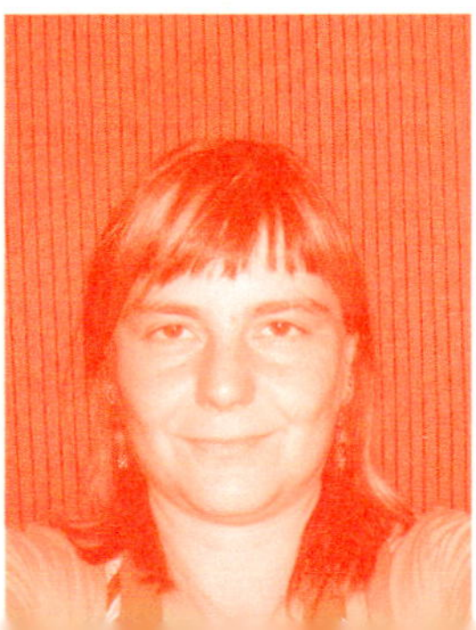

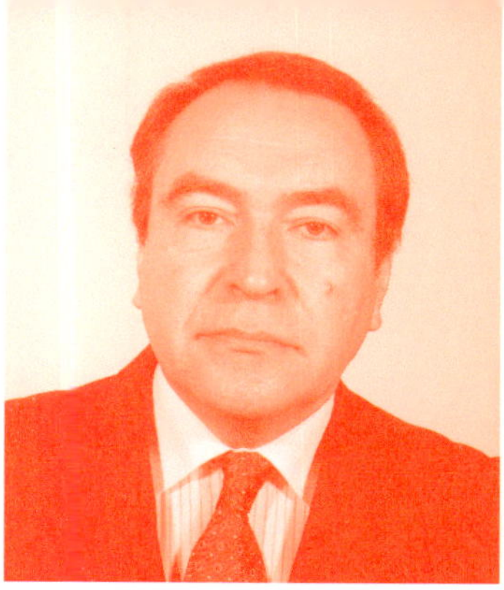
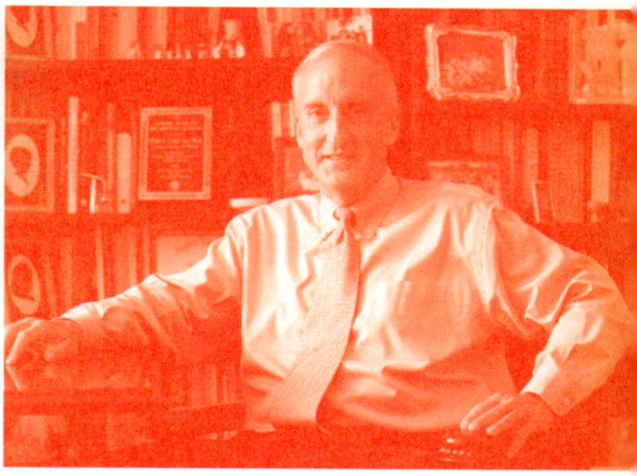
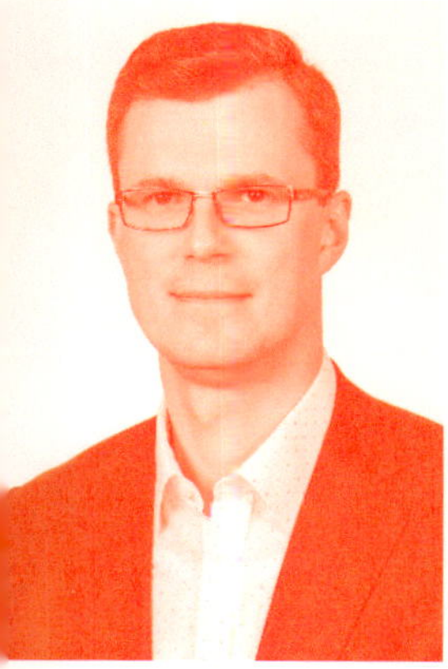
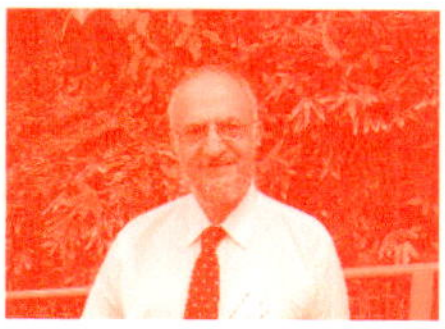
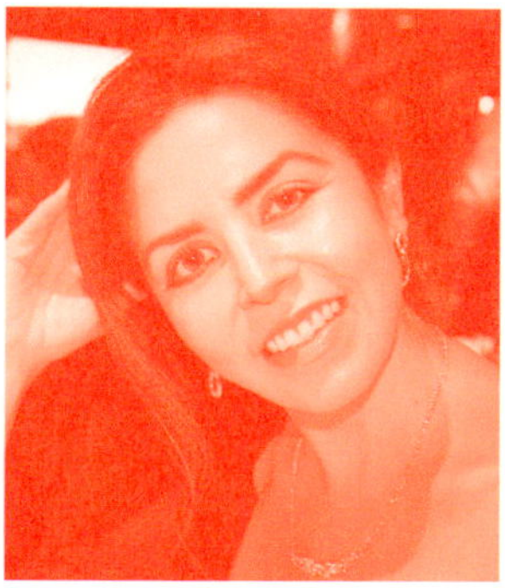

Supporting open minds since 2005

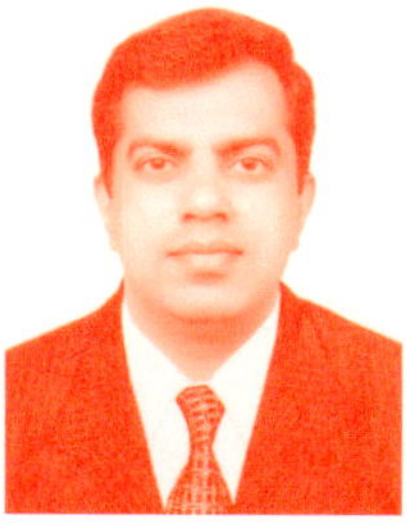
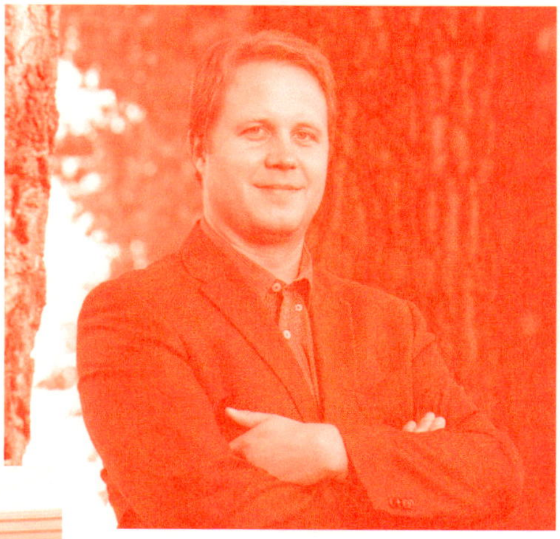
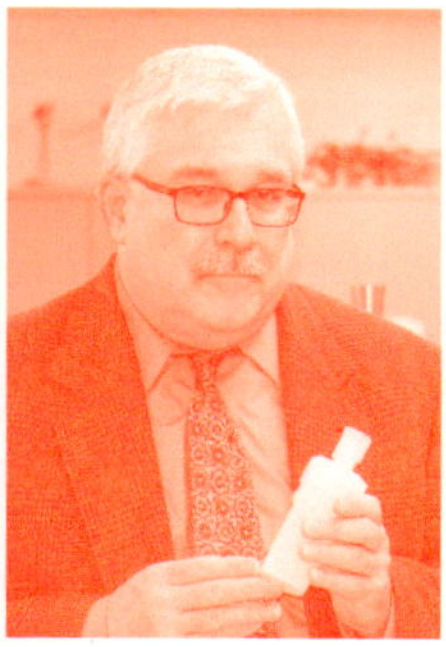
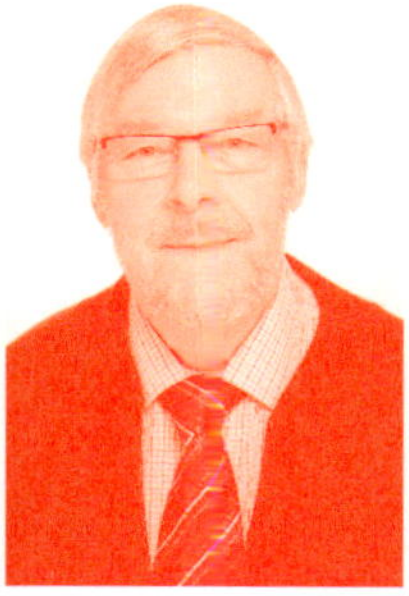
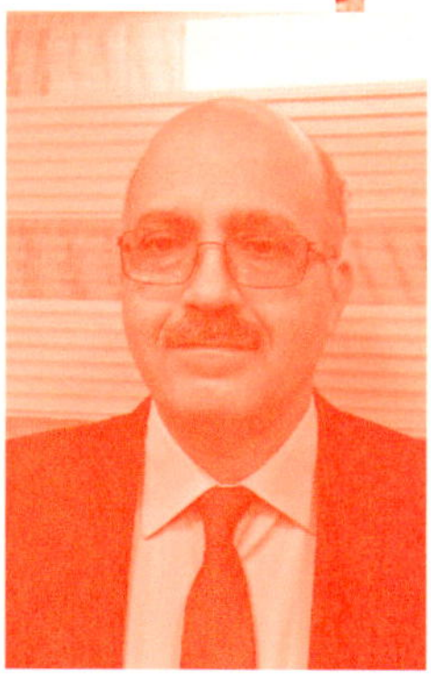
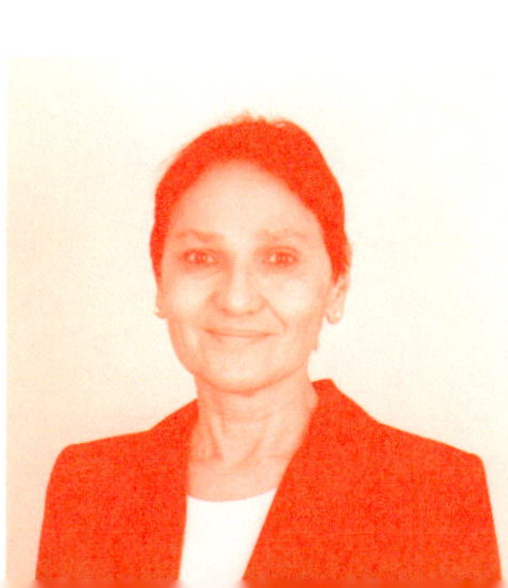
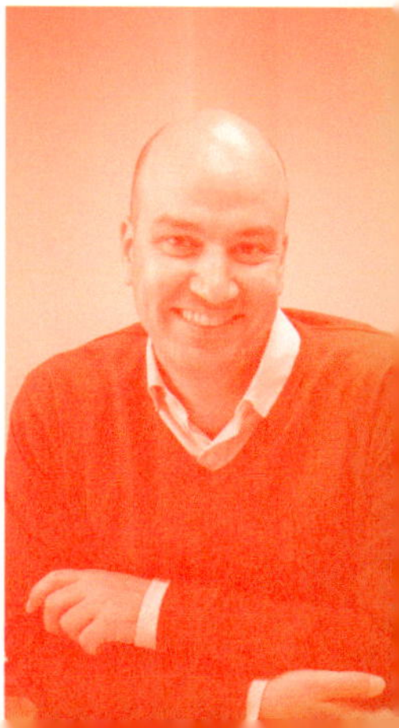

Alginates - Recent Uses of This Natural Polymer
http://dx.doi.org/10.5772/intechopen.77849
Edited by Leonel Pereira

Assistant to the Editor(s): João Cotas

Part of IntechOpen Book Series: Biochemistry, Volume 7
Book Series Editor: Miroslav Blumenberg

Contributors
Takuo Ogihara, Fumiyoshi Kasahara, Yoko Idota, Chihaya Kakinuma, Reza Mohammadi, Jonathan Lakey, Samuel Rodriguez, Rahul Tuli, Ashlyn Wheeler, Amy Nguyen, Jennifer Luong, Michael Alexander, Leonel Pereira, João Cotas, Michail Klontzas, Hicham Drissi, Athanasios Mantalaris, Agnieszka Kaczmarek-Pawelska, Francesca Uberti, Lorenzo Secondini, Ian Stoppa, Mietta Catera, Claudio Molinari, Sudipto Datta, Ranjit Barua, Jonali Das

First published in London, United Kingdom, 2020 by IntechOpen
IntechOpen is the global imprint of INTECHOPEN LIMITED, registered in England and Wales, registration number: 11086078, 7th floor, 10 Lower Thames Street, London, EC3R 6AF, United Kingdom
Printed in Croatia

British Library Cataloguing-in-Publication Data
A catalogue record for this book is available from the British Library

Additional hard and PDF copies can be obtained from orders@intechopen.com

Alginates - Recent Uses of This Natural Polymer
Edited by Leonel Pereira
p. cm.
Print ISBN 978-1-78985-641-5
Online ISBN 978-1-78985-642-2
eBook (PDF) ISBN 978-1-83968-558-3
ISSN 2632-0983

IntechOpen Book Series
Biochemistry
Volume 7

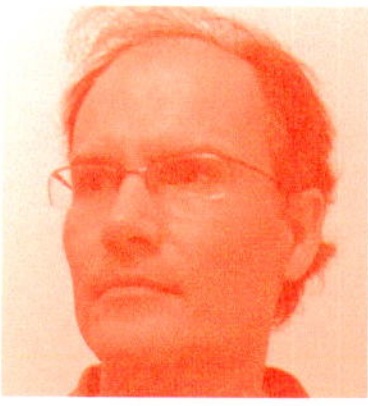

Leonel Pereira has a degree in Biology (Scientific Branch) and a PhD in Biology (specialty Cellular Biology) from the Faculty of Science and Technology of the University of Coimbra, where he is currently a professor. In addition to teaching at this university, he is also an integrated researcher at the Marine and Environmental Sciences Center. His interests are mainly in the areas of marine biodiversity (algae), marine biotechnology (bioactive macroalgal compounds), and marine ecology (environmental assessment). Since 2008, he has been the author and editor of the electronic publication MACOI (www.uc.pt/seaweeds). He is the author of eight books and the editor of five books. He is also the author of 40 book chapters, has published over 41 scientific articles in international journals, and has delivered over 100 lectures and oral communications at international scientific events. He received the award Sea King D. Carlos Prize (18th edition) and the CHOICE Prize—outstanding academic title award 2016 for *Edible Seaweeds of the World*.

Editor of Volume 7: Leonel Pereira
MARE—Marine and Environmental Sciences Centre, Department of Life Sciences, Faculty of Sciences and Technology, University of Coimbra, Portugal

Book Series Editor: Miroslav Blumenberg
NYU Langone Medical Center, New York, USA

Scope of the Series

Biochemistry, the study of chemical transformations occurring within living organisms, impacts all of life sciences, from molecular crystallography and genetics, to ecology, medicine and population biology. Biochemistry studies macromolecules - proteins, nucleic acids, carbohydrates and lipids –their building blocks, structures, functions and interactions. Much of biochemistry is devoted to enzymes, proteins that catalyze chemical reactions, enzyme structures, mechanisms of action and their roles within cells. Biochemistry also studies small signaling molecules, coenzymes, inhibitors, vitamins and hormones, which play roles in the life process. Biochemical experimentation, besides coopting the methods of classical chemistry, e.g., chromatography, adopted new techniques, e.g., X-ray diffraction, electron microscopy, NMR, radioisotopes, and developed sophisticated microbial genetic tools, e.g., auxotroph mutants and their revertants, fermentation etc. More recently, biochemistry embraced the 'big data' omics systems.

Initial biochemical studies have been exclusively analytic: dissecting, purifying and examining individual components of a biological system; in exemplary words of Efraim Racker, (1913 –1991) "Don't waste clean thinking on dirty enzymes." Today however, biochemistry is becoming more agglomerative and comprehensive, setting out to integrate and describe fully a particular biological system. The 'big data' metabolomics can define the complement of small molecules, e.g., in a soil or biofilm sample; proteomics can distinguish all the proteins comprising e.g., serum; metagenomics can identify all the genes in a complex environment e.g., bovine rumen. This Biochemistry Series will address both the current research on biomolecules, and the emerging trends with great promise.

Contents

Preface

Alginates are polysaccharides found in both the intercellular matrix of brown algae and extracellularly covering some species of bacteria. They are widely used by the food industry, giving foods texture properties such as thickening, adhesion, emulsification, gelling, or fullness.

Alginate was characterized in the late nineteenth century and is currently obtained from brown algae collected in coastal regions at sea. Alginate can constitute up to 40% of the dry mass of these algae. Due to its unique properties, for gelling and thickening solutions and acting as immobilization support, the material has become a product of commercial importance. Alginate is widely used in food, cosmetics, and medicines and also finds application in the textile and paper industries. It is currently being used in innovative medical and pharmaceutical applications. Due to its characteristics, it is used as a thickener, emulsion and foam stabilizer, encapsulating agent, gelling agent, film-forming agent, and synthetic fiber, among other possibilities. The alginate currently used is extracted from algae; however, its production by microorganisms allows controlled exploitation of its natural sources.

Alginate is a linear copolymer consisting of the acids α-L-guluronic and β-D-mannuronic with 1–4 bonds. The material varies widely in terms of its proportion between mannuronic (M) and guluronic (G) residues, as well as its sequential structure and degree of polymerization. Thus, the material may have alternating sequences of MG residues and blocks consisting of two or more M or G residues. In many applications for which the material is used it has the ability to form gels whose characteristics depend on the M/G ratio and number of cross-links between polymer chains. Gels are formed in the presence of divalent cations such as Ca^{++} or Mg^{++}, and the presence of G residue sequences is required to exhibit this ability.

This book is divided into the following sections: Introductory section, Pharmaceutical and Medical Uses, and Technological Applications. The first chapter is entitled Introductory Chapter: Alginates—A General Looking. The second section consists of Chapters 2 through 6, respectively: Pharmacological Effects and Utility as a Food Additive of Calcium Alginate; Current Perspective and Advancements of Alginate-based Transplantation Technologies; The Use of Alginate Hydrogels for the Culture of Mesenchymal Stem Cells (MSCs): *In Vitro* and *In Vivo* Paradigms; Alginate-Based Hydrogels in Regenerative Medicine; and Role of Alginates Combined with Natural Extracts to Prevent the Gastric Acid-related Damage. The third and last section consists of two chapters: Importance of Alginate Bio-Ink for 3D Bio-Printing in Tissue Engineering and Regenerative Medicine and Application of Artificial Intelligence in Modern Healthcare Systems.

Acknowledgments: This work has the support of Fundação para a Ciência e Tecnologia, through the strategic project UID/MAR/04292/2019 granted to MARE.

Leonel Pereira and João Cotas
MARE—Marine and Environmental Sciences Centre,
Department of Life Sciences,
Faculty of Sciences and Technology,
University of Coimbra,
Coimbra, Portugal

Section 1

Introduction

Chapter 1

Introductory Chapter: Alginates - A General Overview

Leonel Pereira and João Cotas

1. Introduction

Alginate is an anionic polymer that occurs naturally in brown algae (Phaeophyceae), normally present on the cell walls of these organisms.

Alginate is a structural element designated to be the seaweed's main skeletal compound likewise the cellulose function in terrestrial plants, with the gel located in the cell walls and intercellular matrix conferring the mechanical strength and flexibility necessary to withstand the force of the water in which the seaweed grows [1]. Moreover, this function is reflected in the compositional difference of alginates in different seaweeds.

Alginate varies in composition of the algae from 20 to 60% dry matter, but on average brown algae species has 40% alginate. Alginate in brown algae occurs as gels containing sodium, calcium, strontium, magnesium, and barium ions [2].

Alginate is not a compound exclusively of brown algae because there are bacteria that can also produce alginate, but currently all commercial alginate is extracted from algae biomass [3].

Industrial applications of alginate are linked to the gelation, viscosity, and stabilizer properties that alginate attributes to the solutions and products in which it is present. Normally the alginate is a matrix of alginic acid bound cations, such as calcium, sodium, or magnesium. These ions give greater stability to the alginic acid molecule, where the divalent cations give alginate a very rigid conformation and a stable structure unlike the alginate with monovalent cations.

The biotechnological applications of alginate are based on specific effects of the alginate molecule and its variations depending on the covalent bonds with cations, such as calcium, sodium, or magnesium, and this allows for a great number of applications in several variations of the structure and conformation of the alginate molecule.

Alginates are in vogue for specialized knowledge as a pharmaceutical or biomedical ingredient or as compound for advanced biotechnology, and these investigations are turning to a more detailed study of the properties and structure of alginate, leading to points of scientific innovation that, associated with empirical knowledge, will benefit the traditional techniques of alginate exploitation.

2. History

Alginic acid was first discovered and patented (patent date: 12 January 1881) by the British chemical scientist E. C. C. Stanford, and he continued the work on its discovery, contributing to the elucidation of the chemical structure of alginic acid [3]. The Stanford patent explains how the alginate can be extracted by soaking the algae with water or diluted acid, then extracting with sodium carbonate, and then precipitating the alginate present in the solution by addition of acid [4].

In the second decade of the twentieth century, some scientific groups working separately with alginate found that uronic acid was one of the constituents of alginic acid. Moreover, this discovery led to further study in the years to come. These investigations led to the discovery of D-mannuronic acid in hydrolyzed alginate samples. The nature of the bonds in the uronic acid residues in the alginate was identical to that in the cellulose, through the β 1, 4 bond.

It was only in the 1950s that with the work of Fischer and Dörfel [5], through a chromatographic study of uronic acids, the presence of a different uronic acid from what had been identified was discovered, identifying this new acid with L-guluronic acid. And that acid had a considerable quantity in the sample analyzed, and as such, a quantitative method was developed to determine the two acids present in alginate, mannuronic acid and guluronic acid.

Thereafter, alginate was identified as a binary copolymer composed of residues of guluronic and mannuronic acids, but in general, it was reported that alginic acid was chemically homogeneous and of equal chemical structure, independent of the raw material from which it was extracted.

This principle had to be scientifically proven, and the alginate had to be fractionated chemically from different sources to prove the theory. The development of fractionation techniques was done mainly by Haug [6], who helped the characterization alginate as a block copolymer and in the correlation between the block structure and the physical properties of an alginate with that composition.

3. Chemical structure

The alginate is an unbranched biopolymer family. The alginates consist of 1,4-β-D-mannuronic acid (M) and 1,4 α-L-guluronic acid (G) monomers, with a homogeneous (poly-G, poly-M) or heterogeneous (MG) block composition, which was proven by partial acid hydrolysis. That is, each alginate-producing species may exhibit different alginate compositions and as such differences in the ratio of mannuronic and guluronic acid blocks, varying in composition and sequence [7]. The proportions of the two acids vary from species to species and from different parts of the same seaweed [8].

It was proven that the alginates do not have regular repeating units and that the distribution of the monomers along the polymer chain could not be described; hence the knowledge of the monomeric composition was not sufficient to determine the sequential structure of alginates from diverse species.

Alginate is found in seaweeds as salts of different metals, primarily sodium and calcium, in the intercellular regions and cell walls. Its biological functions in seaweeds are of structural and ion exchange type. Alginate enriched in polymannuronic acid is found in young cell wall tissue and/or intercellular regions, whereas polyguluronic-rich alginate is found in the cell wall having a high affinity for Ca^{2+}, which is mainly responsible for gel strength [9]. Alginate polymer is synthesized in the cytoplasm and then transported to the cell surface [10].

The principal differentiation between algal and bacterial alginates at the molecular level is the presence of O-acetyl groups at C_2 and/or C_3 in the bacterial alginates [11].

4. Alginate extraction

The extraction methodology of alginate is recurring on the transforming of the insoluble mixture of the alginic acid salts prevenient of the cell wall in a soluble alginate salt, which is naturally recommended for aqueous high-affinity polysaccharide obtained from the main species of brown algae (e.g., Fucales and Laminariales). The industry uses brown seaweeds mainly from the genus *Macrocystis*, *Laminaria* (**Figure 1a**), *Lessonia*, *Ascophyllum*, *Alaria*, *Ecklonia*, *Eisenia*, *Nereocystis*, *Sargassum*, *Cystoseira*, and *Fucus* (**Figure 1b**), with *Macrocystis pyrifera* (**Figure 1c**) and *Ascophyllum nodosum* (**Figure 1d**) being the principal resources utilized.

Various species are harvested, and some are even cultivated offshore (e.g., *Laminaria* and *Alaria* (**Figure 1e**)) for alginate production, between southern and northern hemispheres. The species used are generally harvested from natural resources. China and some northern hemisphere countries, however, cultivate these species, which is an expensive way of alginate production. In this case, *Laminaria* is mostly used as food, and if surplus amounts are cultivated, then it can be used for alginate production.

Brown seaweeds that grow in cold water and those growing at a temperature up to 20°C are more used because they have more alginic acid content than the brown seaweeds found in more warm waters. And due to more turbulent waters, the seaweeds produce more content than the same species in calmer waters [12].

The alginic acid appears in the seaweeds as an insoluble mixed salt. To extract it, it is necessary to convert the alginic acid into its soluble salt forms such as sodium or potassium [12]. The alginate is made alternately insoluble and soluble in solvent by ion exchange reactions to separate out from the other constituents of algae. As large molecules must diffuse out from the plant tissues, the seaweed is preferably reduced to small particles as a preliminary step. Therefore, the first step is to wash (dry, if necessary) and mill the seaweed. Alginate isolation is essentially an ion exchange process, and alginate is brought into solution as sodium alginate by treating it with a strong alkali, after a pre-treatment with hydrochloric acid before the extraction with sodium carbonate [13, 14]. There are several methods to separate the alginate from other soluble substances from the crude alginate extract solution.

For example, addition of alcohol [2] would precipitate out sodium alginate. Adding a solution of calcium chloride with good stirring would precipitate out calcium alginate, whereas adding hydrochloric acid would precipitate out alginic acid.

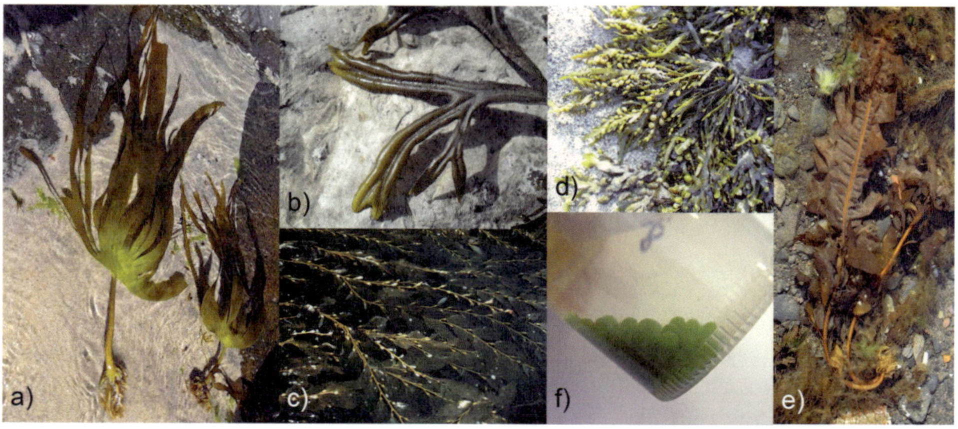

Figure 1.
(a) Laminaria ochroleuca from Ínsua beach, afife, north of Portugal; (b) Fucus ceranoides from mondego river estuary (coordinates: 40° 7'31.39"N, 8°46'15.76"W), center-north of Portugal; (c) Macrocystis pyrifera; (d) Ascophyllum nodosum from Praia do norte, Viana Do Castelo, north of Portugal; (e) Alaria esculenta from Eskifjördur, Iceland; (f) Chlorella vulgaris immobilized in calcium alginate gel beads. Original images: (a, d, and e) University of Coimbra (MACOI), (b and f) João cotas images in public domain: (c) Shane Anderson.

The extraction of alginate is done by mild acid treatments that remove undesirable compounds (normally, hydrochloric acid) and modify the cell wall alginate into alginic acid to obtain the best extract efficacy because the intercellular mucilage has been regarded as the principal site of alginic acid [15]. The alginic acid is recovered as a soluble sodium form by neutralizing with sodium carbonate or sodium hydroxide. The insoluble residue is removed by filtration, flotation, or centrifugation, and the soluble alginate is precipitated by conversion into alginic acid or calcium/sodium alginate. The alginic acid is then converted into the required counter ion by neutralization with appropriate hydroxides or chlorites. The difference in the alginate recovery process depends on the source and structure of constituents of alginate [13].

5. Alginates as valuable resource

Alginates are used in the food, cosmetic, paper, agricultural, pharmaceutical, and biomedical industries and in other various industries; some are now starting to apply the alginates. The alginates overall are the main seaweed polymer, in terms of quantities, used by industry. There are different purity classes of alginates ready to apply for different uses; with that, the price of alginates varies according to the purity state and applications on the industry. For instance, the alimentary grade sodium alginate is priced at USD 6.5 and 11.0/kg, while pharmaceutical grade is valued at USD 13 and 15.5/kg. In Asia, more specifically in the Korean peninsula and in Japan, *Saccharina japonica* (formerly *Laminaria japonica*) has a big demand which resulted in a higher price, which resulted in the introduction of buying alginates from other countries [16]. Alginate market is expected to grow annually between 2 and 3%. The uses of alginate in the industry, such as textile printing, account for nearly half of the global market. On the biomedical, medical, and pharmaceutical industries, it has an implication of nearly 20% of the global market, and it is expected to grow between 2 and 4% in the global market, lying on the applications of alginic acid derivatives in wound healing and regular basis innovations and developments in controlled-release technologies. Paper industry only reports to nearly 5% of the global market [17].

Alginates are mainly used as thickeners and stabilizers in the food, pharmaceutical, and cosmetic industries, because they are easy to use, has a low cost, are well tolerated in the human, and can be easily modified for determined objective and in the different fields.

Today, the global seaweed industry is worth more than USD 6 billion per annum (approximately 12 million tons per annum in volume) of which 85% is in the food area for human consumption. Seaweed-derived polysaccharides (carrageenan, agar, and alginates) make up almost 40% of the world's hydrocolloid market [18].

The global alginate market size was valued at USD 624.0 million in 2016. The demand for alginates in the food industry will be increasing by consumption of frozen desserts, ice creams, beer, and yogurt; with that, it is anticipated to push a salient market growth of alginate value and use.

The application of the alginates in the food industry is permitted and regulated by the major regulatory agencies including the FDA and European Commission, which stimulates the high interest in alginate. The increasing of food industry in Asia, due to the growth in habitants, is expected to run a higher demand of alginate in that area. Therefore, this alginates-based products acceptance by the manufacturing industries is expected to growth, such as biomedical industry and its high demand for alginate with high quality. The product is mainly used in the pharmaceutical industry for the production of controlled-release drugs due to superior product performance [19].

Corporations in the market devote to the investigation and development of new advanced product grades to captivate costumers. Extraordinary financing by national governments and alginate industries on route to the growth of seaweed processing is predicted to help the alginate-based industry's expansion and success. Nevertheless, such high search for alginate can have as outcome a limited raw material availability, and the alginate industry is now evaluating the production of alginate with seaweeds of aquaculture (mainly offshore, at this moment in the North Atlantic Area and China).

There is a large market for any brown seaweed that has an alginate of medium to high viscosity or high gel strength [20].

5.1 Agricultural applications

Alginate present in the brown algae (in the form of alginic acid) constituted a functional element of the traditional fertilizers, allowing the water retention in the soils. So, the principal function of alginate on agricultural area was as a soil conditioner. Being a superabsorbent (SAP) or water-retaining material is an advantage of alginate. They are natural materials that can absorb large amounts of water, as much as hundreds of times their own mass. These alginates are generally known in agriculture as nonionic or ionic moisture-holding hydrogels for increasing soil water retention, which is a basic soil property.

The reservation of moisture or water in the soil is the major process consequence in which all plantations depend. The large pore spaces in arenaceous soils restrain the soil from holding water, and the soil dries out regularly, and precious nutrients wash away past the plant roots. The inclusion of alginate can solve the lack of retention of water and raise nutrient disponibility. High-capacity absorbents definitely can upsurge the water-retention capacity in such soils.

Superabsorbents (SAP) in agricultural areas have been designed and developed to provoke an enrichment of the abiotic properties of soil by rising their water-retention ability, developing a better water usage efficiency, enhancing soil permeability and infiltration rates, contributing to lower the irrigation frequency, lowering the compaction shift, preventing erosion and water drainage, enhancing plant performance, increasing soil aeration, lowering the dissolution of fertilizers, developing a better adsorption capacity or enhancing the uptake of some nutrient elements by the plants, and provoking a raise of the microbial activity [21].

The alginate of seaweed directly suppresses the pathogens [22]. Indeed, alginate pellets developed as carrier material for biocontrol agents have been reported to reduce multiplication of *Rhizoctonia* (fungi) disease in potato [23], while incorporation of *Ascophyllum nodosum* extract into the planting medium caused delay and reduced incidence of *Verticillium* (fungi) wilt of pepper plants [24]. Therefore, it's proven that alginates are involved in host defense mechanisms [25]. Of particular interest in agriculture are those that elicit defensive responses resulting in protection against pathogens or insect damage [26].

In other cases, the alginate will have other particular function, as the main characteristic of alginate as product principal emulsifier and to delivery control of actives ingredients in agricultural field. The active ingredient is mixed with alginates for their safer, easier, and more accurate handling as well as for their effective application in the field and, at the same time, preventing the immediate release of the active ingredient, so the main drawback associated with these formulations can be avoided. These alginate-based systems are able to deliver the active ingredient gradually for a long period of time in a specified target with a desired rate [27–29]. The controlled-release systems do not release the active ingredient at once; this technique therefore lowers the pesticide residues in soil and thus reduces the direct effect of pesticide. After their degradation, these are helpful as compost in the field [30].

Alginate is also used as an inoculant carrier for plant growth-promoting bacteria [31, 32] and for bacteria with biodegradation ability [33].

5.2 Biomedical applications

The conventional role of alginate in the biomedical area includes being used as thickening, gel-forming, and stabilizing agents, as alginate can play a significant role in controlled-release drug products. But the main use of alginate in the biomedical area is actually in hydrogel form, used in the wound healing [34], drug delivery, and tissue engineering applications. Alginate hydrogels are biocompatible and structurally identical to the macromolecular-based components in the human body and can regularly be convoyed into the body by minor invasive techniques of administration to the select human body [35].

In this area, there is a need that the alginate used and tested is pure as maximum as possible, because the impurities will compromise the biocompatibility of the biomaterial with alginate [36].

The utmost captivating characteristics of alginate for the biomedical applications involve the natural biocompatibility, mild gelation conditions, and easy adaptation to assemble alginate derivatives with new properties and characteristics. Alginate has a safe clinical sheet for biomedical applications as a wound dressing material and pharmaceutical component and has been harmlessly inserted in a wide range of utilizations.

The conception of new biomaterials is centralized on the resemblance in the functions of the extracellular matrices of body tissues, as these can manage the host feedback/responses in an accurate behavior, and materials derived from natural sources have gained a lot of interest, mainly because of their inherent biocompatibility. At this moment, alginate and its derivatives are one of the best chemically known biopolymers in the world, and it has been extensively investigated and used for many biomedical applications, due to its biocompatibility, low toxicity, relatively low cost, and mild gelation by addition of divalent cations such as Ca^{2+} [37].

The great challenge in this area is complementing the physical feature of alginate gels with specific use in a precise utilization. Taking in consideration the great range of different possible cross-linking approaches, employing molecules with diversified chemical structures, molecular weights, and cross-linking capabilities will usually turnout gels applicable for specifics different types of application [36].

Alginate-based wound dressings keep the physiologically humid microenvironment, lowering the risks of a bacterial infection at the wound location and promoting an easy wound healing. Drug compounds, from small chemical drugs to macromolecular proteins, can be liberated from alginate gels in a skillful way, revolving around in the cross-links types and cross-linking methodology applied.

The therapy of acute and chronic wounds is a major need in various areas of medicine, and alginate-based wound dressings have various beneficial properties. Traditional wound dressings, such as gauze, provide principally a good barrier property—maintaining the wound dry by granting the evaporation of wound exudates and preventing the passage of pathogens into the wound [38]. In the opposite way, the modern dressings, likewise the alginate dressings, contribute to a moist wound environment and aid an easy wound healing [39].

New wound dressing types with alginate that are more functional and bioactive have been studied and developed up to this date.

Alginate gels are additionally an excellent compound for cell transplantation in the tissue engineering area. The main objective of tissue engineering was to develop and produce man-made tissue and organ replacements for patients who suffer the loss or failure of an organ or tissue [40]. In this field, hydrogels are used to deliver cells to the specific location, providing an area for new tissue formation and, moreover, controlling the structure and function of the engineered tissue [41].

Even with recent developments in the area, the treatment of bone injuries is restricting because of the poor healing and complex bone healing system. In this case, alginate gels have been tested with success in bone regeneration by delivery of osteoinductive factors, bone-forming cells, or a mixture of both [42].

Alginate gels have been described to be effective for transplanting chondrogenic cells to recover damaged cartilage in animal models [43].

Alginate gels are also being actively investigated for their ability to mediate the regeneration and engineering of a variety of other tissues and organs, including skeletal muscle, nerve, the pancreas, and the liver. Actual plans for skeletal muscle regeneration involve the cell transplantation, growth factor delivery, or a combination of both approaches [44, 45], and alginate gels have been described as potential hypothesis in these strategies.

Alginate derivatives containing cell-adhesive peptides have been gaining significant attraction in the last years. These derivatives are normally prepared by chemically including peptides as side chains, applying carbodiimide chemistry to connect via the carboxylic groups of the sugar residues. Considering that alginate intrinsically do not have mammalian cell adhesiveness, pertinent ligands are essential to develop and manage cellular interactions, principally for cell culture [36].With that, the alginate gels are now being utilized much more as a model system for mammalian cell culture in this field. And one of the advantages is that the gels can be adapted to 2D or more physiologically relevant 3D culture systems.

The absence of mammalian cell receptors joined with the low protein adsorption to the gels enables the utilization of these materials in many ways as an ideal blank slate, with highly specific and quantitative modes for cell adhesion that can be incorporated. Also development demonstrated with in vitro studies can be readily translated in vivo, because of the inherent biocompatibility and easy introduction of alginate into the body [36].

Alginate hydrogels have been widely investigated to date in many drug delivery applications, due to their adjustable swelling properties in response to temperature changes, leading to on-demand modulation of drug release from the gels [46].

Alginate is a nondegradable material in mammals, as the mammals do not have enzymes (i.e., alginase) that can break the alginate chains, but ionically cross-linked alginate-base gels can be disassociated by release of the divalent ions cross-linking the gel into the surrounding media. Despite the gel dissolution, the average molecular weights of many commercially available alginates are higher than the renal clearance threshold of the kidneys, and presumably dissolved alginate isn't removed from the body with 100% efficiency [47].

Alginate has also been greatly explored in plenty drug delivery systems merged with chitosan, and this blend forms ionic complexes. Chitosan is a derivative of chitin [48].

Alginate is an attractive and exceptional contender for the protein drug delivery systems, considering that alginate-based materials/gels can incorporate proteins [49, 50]. The delivery in this scenario can be easily exploited by modifying the degradation rate of the gels [50].

Also, alginate can serve as an agent against heavy metal poisoning, and it is proven that it can be an effective coadjuvant in the case of food poisoning [51].

On the medical side, there has been an increment of interest to use alginate as a pharmaceutical ingredient to treat some diseases or health problems:

Diabetes—This bioactivity is related to the hypoglycemic activity from alginate [52].

Cholesterol—The alginate on the assay in article [52] with rats provides interesting results, with cholesterol excretion from the rats and hypocholesterolemic effect from alginate.

Obesity—The capacity of alginate to swell and so occupy space on the stomach of the patient provides a satiety effect which can help people lose weight and provide a management tool for the medical personnel [53];

Digestive tract problems—The alginate is used as dietary fiber and can regulate the intestinal tract.

5.3 Bioremediation applications

Environmental bioremediation is a profitable and promising technology, which can lead to complete mineralization of organic pollution. Bioaugmentation (introduction of selected microorganisms to supplement indigenous populations) is one of the bioremediation approaches [54]. Entrapment in alginate gel is a widely used approach for immobilization of microorganisms to improve their viability (**Figure 1f**) [55].

Alginate is a natural chelating agent and a bio-adsorbent of heavy metals in aqueous solution; it has high affinity and binding capacity for metal ions and, thus, is widely used as a heavy metal adsorbent for environmental protection [56]. Alginate-clay composites are suitable for environmental remediation as sorbents of heavy metals [57] and persistent organic pollutants [58].

5.4 Cosmetic applications

Alginates are an omnipresent ingredient of cosmetics. They usually are utilized as emulsifiers, consistency enhancers, and thickening agents in cosmetic formulas, forming a moisture-retaining surface film. They can have some kind of active effect, such as skin protection, because they retain water and maintain the skin rehydrated [59].

Alginates are water-insoluble; however, they can swell, as mentioned before. Thus, they are like hyaluronic acid, so they can absorb more water as much as several hundreds of times its weight.

They are used in hand jellies and lotions, ointment bases, pomades and other similar preparations, greaseless creams, dentifrices, and other products that became more green and environmentally friendly [60, 61].

Alginate has also been described as an anti-oxidative agent and can be applied to prevent skin aging and cutaneous disorders. Additionally, antioxidants can help to maintain the organoleptic properties of cosmetic products by inhibiting lipid oxidation, thus avoiding changes in appearance, odor, and flavor [62].

5.5 Food applications

Alginates are commonly used in the food industry as natural additives; they have codes from the European Union as food additives, and these codes vary with the ion type associated with alginic acid [15, 63].

European codes for alginates are as follows: alginic acid, E400; sodium alginate, E401; potassium alginate, E402; ammonium alginate, E403; calcium alginate, E404; and propylene glycol alginate, E405.

Seaweed polysaccharide applications in food industries are based mainly on their stabilizing, emulsifying, and gel-forming ability. They are widely used as food additives in jams, jellies, ice creams, dairy products, etc., to improve and stabilize the structure of food.

Water-in-oil emulsions likewise the mayonnaise and the salad fillings are less liable to fractionate toward their original oil and water phases if thickened with alginate. When the emulsion is acidic, the sodium alginate will precipitate into insoluble alginic acid forms; to resolve this problem, propylene glycol alginate (PGA) is used for acidic emulsions, because this compound is stable in mild acid conditions [63].

The advantage of alginate in the food industry is that humans do not have enzymes to break the molecule; therefore, alginate behaves as a dietary fiber, enhancing the satiety and reducing the food intake of humans, lowering the energy intake by human, and preventing obesity [53].

5.6 Dental medicine applications

Hydrocolloids were the first elastic materials to be used in the dental field, and their results are fundamental to form a first "idea" about the patient's oral health status.

The alginate is used as irreversible footprint compound to emulate a footprint faithfully, giving details in a high-definition footprint although there is an existence of undercuts.

The main alginate advantages are the fact that they are low cost, do not react adversely on the patient, and can be easily manipulated and that the technique can be performed within a short period of time and has simple execution, lack of instrumentation, and high-definition footprint, even with the presence of undercuts, in a single-step methodology.

Alginate picking reaction is a chemical reaction of irreversible precipitation; therefore they cannot return in soluble form using physical means, such as temperature, as with reversible hydrocolloids [64].

5.7 Other areas of alginate application

Packaging dominates the waste generated from plastics. Since the European Union synthetic plastic ban, alginate is one of the most suitable alternatives to fabricate packaging material due to their nontoxicity, biodegradability, and derivability from renewable natural resources.

With the bibliography analysis, it can be resumed that additives such as nonmaterial and antimicrobial compounds can improve various characteristics of the films and the packaging with antimicrobial activity is highly desirable in films to improve the shelf life of packed food products [56].

In textile printing, alginates are used as thickeners for the paste containing the dye. These pastes may be applied to the fabric by the use of either screen or roller printing equipment. These combine chemically with cellulose in the fabric. Alginates don't interact with the dyes; also they can be washed out of the finalized textile and are considered the first-rate thickeners to the reactive dyes [20].

The principal alginate application in the paper industry is in surface sizing. Alginate is mixed with starch sizing giving a smooth uninterrupted film and a surface with less fluffing. The oil resistance derivate from alginate films allows a size with improved greaseproof and oil-resistant properties. This can enhance the gloss obtained with high gloss inks.

If papers or boards need to be waxed, alginate in the size maintains the wax at the surface.

Alginates provide a better coating runnability than other similar compounds/products, specifically in hot, on-machine coating applications.

They are also exceptional film formers and enhance the ink printability and resistance. In the size, the normal mixture of alginate is 5–10% of the total weight of starch. Alginate is used in the starch adhesives to form corrugated boards, because it stabilizes the viscosity of the adhesive and allows control of its rate of penetration [20].

The applications of alginates in new areas has proven the multi-role capacity of alginates, such as supportive agent for silicon nanopowder to yield a stable battery anode that possesses reversible capacity eight times higher than that of the state-of-the-art graphitic anodes. Improved performance characteristics prevent the dramatic volume changes during electrochemical alloying and de-alloying with Li, which typically leads to rapid anode degradation [65].

In the specialized clothing industry, the alginate anti-fire capacity was proven to be effective. The new alginate-based materials are showing enormous potential to be applied in building insulation materials and textile industry [66–68]

6. Conclusion

Humans use seaweed since the inception of civilization due to its medicinal properties and other properties, such as manure for the infertile soils. There is also a long history of alginate usage in foods as additives and as emulsifying, gelling, and stabilizing agents. And those characteristics open new areas and industries where alginate can be harnessed and used with success.

In bioremediation, the alginate can act as heavy metal chelating agent and support new technology to rehabilitate the degraded ecosystems.

This function can also serve as medical support to patients poisoned with heavy metals.

Although it was discovered in 1881, one of the main characteristics of alginate was used for a long time without notice: this was as soil conditioner by Europeans and other people since the Bronze Age.

Alginate is one of the easiest and low-cost natural polymers, and because of these particularities, alginate is the most researched polymer among all seaweed polysaccharides. Alginate advantages are now being explored for innovations on other areas, and that is improving the knowledge about alginates.

On the biomedical area, the alginate-based compounds/products will be on the front line of the new emergent methods and techniques evolving the human and animal health in various medical areas. This is happening now with wound dressings and the addition of regeneration factors in the alginate-based ones.

It is believed that with the new demand of natural polymers to substitute synthetic polymers, the alginate from various forms will be harnessed and will gain new types of applications in the industries that work with polymers. That demand is now sorting effects with the increment of investigation and development of new techniques and methods to work with alginate and its subforms, such as alginate-nanoclay complexes.

Acknowledgements

This work had the support of Fundação para a Ciência e Tecnologia (FCT), through the strategic project UID/MAR/04292/2019 granted to MARE. This work also received funding from the European Structural and Investment Funds through the COMPETE Programme and from National Funds through Fundação para a Ciência e a Tecnologia (FCT) under the program grant SAICTPAC/0019/2015.

This work is also co-financed by the European Regional Development Fund through the Interreg Atlantic Area Programme, under the project NASPA.

Conflict of interest

The authors declare no conflict of interest.

Author details

Leonel Pereira and João Cotas*
Marine and Environmental Sciences Centre (MARE), Department of Life Sciences, Faculty of Sciences and Technology, University of Coimbra, Coimbra, Portugal

*Address all correspondence to: jcotas@gmail.com

References

[1] Sudha PN, editor. Industrial Applications of Marine Biopolymers. Boca Raton: CRC Press; 2017. 626 p

[2] Haug A, Smidsrød O. Strontium–calcium selectivity of alginates. Nature. 1967;**215**(5102):757

[3] Draget KI, Smidsrød O, Skjåk-Bræk G. Alginates from algae. Biopolymers. 2005:1-30

[4] Hoagland DR, Lieb LL. The complex carbohydrates and forms of Sulphur in marine algae of the Pacific coast. The Journal of Biological Chemistry. 1915;**23**(1):287-297

[5] Fischer FG, Dörfel H. Die Polyuronsäuren der braunalgen (kohlenhydrate der algen I). Hoppe-Seyler's Zeitschrift für Physiologische Chemie. 1955;**302**:186-203

[6] Draget KI, Skjåk Bræk G, Smidsrød O. Alginic acid gels: The effect of alginate chemical composition and molecular weight. Carbohydrate Polymers. 1994;**25**(1):31-38

[7] Szekalska M, Puciłowska A, Szymańska E, Ciosek P, Winnicka K. Alginate: Current use and future perspectives in pharmaceutical and biomedical applications. International Journal of Polymer Science. 2016;**2016**:1-17

[8] Haug A, Larsen B, Smidsrød O. Uronic acid sequence in alginate from different sources. Carbohydrate Research. 1974;**32**(2):217-225

[9] Arunkumar K. Extraction, isolation, and characterization of alginate. In: Sudha PN, editor. Industrial Applications of Marine Biopolymers. Boca Raton: CRC Press; 2017. pp. 19-35

[10] Abe K, Sakamoto T, Sasaki SF, Nisizawa K. In vivo studies of the synthesis of alginic acid in ishige okamurai. Botanica Marina. 1973;**16**(4):229-234

[11] Skjåk-Bræk G, Grasdalen H, Larsen B. Monomer sequence and acetylation pattern in some bacterial alginates. Carbohydrate Research. 1986;**154**(1):239-250

[12] Clare K. Algin. Industrial Gums. 1993:105-143

[13] McHugh DJ. Production and Utilization of Products from Commercial Seaweeds. FAO Fisheries Technical Paper No. 288. Vol. 1891987

[14] Sime WJ. Alginates. In: Harris P, editor. Food Gels. Dordrecht: Springer Netherlands; 1990. pp. 53-78

[15] Pereira L, Gheda SF, Ribeiro-Claro PJ. Analysis by vibrational spectroscopy of seaweed polysaccharides with potential use in food, pharmaceutical, and cosmetic industries. International Journal of Carbohydrate Chemistry. 2013;**2013**(vi):1-7

[16] Gillespie RD, Critchley AT. Phenology of *Sargassum spp.* (sargassaceae, phaeophyta) from Reunion rocks, KwaZulu-Natal, South Africa. Hydrobiologia. 1999;**398-399**(April):201-210

[17] Kraan S. Algal polysaccharides, novel applications and outlook. In: Chang C-F, editor. Carbohydrates—Comprehensive Studies on Glycobiology and Glycotechnology. InTech; 2012. pp. 489-532. DOI: 10.5772/51572

[18] Ferdouse F, Holdt SL, Smith R, Murúa P, Yang Z. The global status of seaweed production, trade and utilization. FAO Globefish Research Program. 2018;**124**:120

[19] Alginate Market Analysis By Type (High G, High M), By Product (Sodium Alginate, Calcium Alginate, Potassium Alginate, Propylene Glycol Alginate), By Application, And Segment Forecasts. 2018-2025 [Internet]. 2017. p. 127. Available from: https://www.grandviewresearch.com/industry-analysis/alginate-market

[20] McHugh DJ. A guide to the seaweed industry. In: FAO Fisheries Technical Paper 441. 2003. pp. 1-105

[21] Abd El-Rehim HA. Characterization and possible agricultural application of polyacrylamide/sodium alginate crosslinked hydrogels prepared by ionizing radiation. Journal of Applied Polymer Science. 2006;**101**(6):3572-3580

[22] Sultana V, Baloch GN, Ambreen AJ, Rajput Tariq M, Ehteshamul-Haque S. Comparative efficacy of a red alga *Solieria robusta*, chemical fertilizers and pesticides in managing the root diseases and growth of soybean. Pakistan Journal of Botany. 2011;**43**(1):1-6

[23] Jacobs H, Gray SN, Crump DH. Interactions between nematophagous fungi and consequences for their potential as biological agents for the control of potato cyst nematodes. Mycological Research. 2003;**107**(Pt 1):47-56

[24] Jayaraj J, Wan A, Rahman M, Punja ZK. Seaweed extract reduces foliar fungal diseases on carrot. Crop Protection. 2008;**27**(10):1360-1366

[25] Craigie JS. Seaweed extract stimuli in plant science and agriculture. Journal of Applied Phycology. 2011;**23**(3):371-393

[26] Chatzissavvidis C, Therios I. Role of algae in agriculture. In: Pomin VH, editor. Seaweeds: Agricultural Uses, Biological and Antioxidant Agents. New York: Nova Science Publishers; 2014. pp. 1-37

[27] Nair R, Varghese SH, Nair BG, Maekawa T, Yoshida Y, Kumar DS. Nanoparticulate material delivery to plants. Plant Science. 2010;**179**(3):154-163

[28] Gogos A, Knauer K, Bucheli TD. Nanomaterials in plant protection and fertilization: Current state, foreseen applications, and research priorities. Journal of Agricultural and Food Chemistry. 2012;**60**(39):9781-9792

[29] Campos EVR, de Oliveira JL, Fraceto LF. Applications of controlled release Systems for Fungicides, herbicides, acaricides, nutrients, and plant growth hormones: A review. Advanced Science, Engineering and Medicine. 2014;**6**(4):373-387

[30] Kumar S, Bhanjana G, Sharma A, Sidhu MC, Dilbaghi N. Synthesis, characterization and on field evaluation of pesticide loaded sodium alginate nanoparticles. Carbohydrate Polymers. 2014;**101**:1061-1067

[31] Bashan Y. Alginate beads as synthetic inoculant carriers for slow release of bacteria that affect plant growth. Applied and Environmental Microbiology. 1986;**51**(5):1089-1098

[32] Trivedi P, Pandey A, Palni LMS. Carrier-based preparations of plant growth-promoting bacterial inoculants suitable for use in cooler regions. World Journal of Microbiology and Biotechnology. 2005;**21**(6-7):941-945

[33] Li H, Li P, Hua T, Zhang Y, Xiong X, Gong Z. Bioremediation of contaminated surface water by immobilized *Micrococcus roseus*. Environmental Technology. 2005;**26**(8):931-940

[34] Pielesz A, Machnicka A, Sarna E. Antibacterial activity and scanning electron microscopy (sem) examination of alginate-based films and wound dressings. Ecological Chemistry and Engineering S-Chemia I Inzynieria Ekologiczna S. 2011;**18**(2):197-210

[35] Sakiyama-Elbert S, Hubbell J. Functional biomaterials: Design of Novel Biomaterials. Annual Review of Materials Research. 2001;**31**(1):183-201

[36] Lee KY, Mooney DJ. Alginate: Properties and biomedical applications. Progress in Polymer Science. 2012;**37**(1):106-126

[37] Gombotz WR, Wee S. Protein release from alginate matrices. Advanced Drug Delivery Reviews. 1998;**31**(3):267-285

[38] Boateng JS, Matthews KH, Stevens HNE, Eccleston GM. Wound healing dressings and drug delivery systems: A review. Journal of Pharmaceutical Sciences. 2008;**97**(8):2892-2923

[39] Queen D, Orsted H, Sanada H, Sussman G. A dressing history. International Wound Journal. 2004;**1**(1):59-77

[40] Langer R, Vacanti J. Tissue engineering. Science. 1993;**260**(5110):920-926

[41] Lee KY, Mooney DJ. Hydrogels for tissue engineering. Chemical Reviews. 2001;**101**(7):1869-1879

[42] Kolambkar YM, Dupont KM, Boerckel JD, Huebsch N, Mooney DJ, Hutmacher DW, et al. An alginate-based hybrid system for growth factor delivery in the functional repair of large bone defects. Biomaterials. 2011;**32**(1):65-74

[43] Thornton AJ, Alsberg E, Albertelli M, Mooney DJ. Shape-defining scaffolds for minimally invasive tissue engineering. Transplantation. 2004;**77**(12):1798-1803

[44] Saxena AK, Marler J, Benvenuto M, Willital GH, Vacanti JP. Skeletal muscle tissue engineering using isolated myoblasts on synthetic biodegradable polymers: Preliminary studies. Tissue Engineering. 1999;**5**(6):525-531

[45] Levenberg S, Rouwkema J, Macdonald M, Garfein ES, KohaneDS, DarlandDC, etal. Engineering vascularized skeletal muscle tissue. Nature Biotechnology. 2005;**23**(7):879-884

[46] Roy D, Cambre JN, Sumerlin BS. Future perspectives and recent advances in stimuli-responsive materials. Progress in Polymer Science. 2010;**35**(1-2): 278-301

[47] Al-Shamkhani A, Duncan R. Radioiodination of alginate via covalently-bound tyrosinamide allows monitoring of its fate in vivo. Journal of Bioactive and Compatible Polymers. 1995;**10**(1):4-13

[48] Sandford PA, Steinnes A. In: Shalaby SW, McCormick CL, Butler GB, editors. Water-Soluble PolymersBiomedical Applications of High-Purity Chitosan. Vol. 467. Washington, DC: American Chemical Society; 1991. pp. 430-445

[49] Lee KY, Peters MC, Mooney DJ. Comparison of vascular endothelial growth factor and basic fibroblast growth factor on angiogenesis in SCID mice. Journal of Controlled Release. 2003;**87**(1-3):49-56

[50] Silva EA, Mooney DJ. Effects of VEGF temporal and spatial presentation on angiogenesis. Biomaterials. 2010;**31**(6):1235-1241

[51] Eliaz I, Weil E, Wilk B. Integrative medicine and the role of modified citrus

pectin/alginates in heavy metal chelation and detoxification - five case reports. Forschende Komplementärmedizin. 2007;**14**(6):358-364

[52] Mariya V, Ravindran VS. Biomedical and pharmacological significance of marine macro algae-review. Indian Journal of Marine Sciences. 2013;**42**(5):527-537

[53] Brown EM, Allsopp PJ, Magee PJ, Gill CI, Nitecki S, Strain CR, et al. Seaweed and human health. Nutrition Reviews. 2014;**72**(3):205-216

[54] Hassanshahian M, Emtiazi G, Caruso G, Cappello S. Bioremediation (bioaugmentation/biostimulation) trials of oil polluted seawater: A mesocosm simulation study. Marine Environmental Research. 2014;**95**:28-38

[55] Zommere Ž, Nikolajeva V. Immobilization of bacterial association in alginate beads for bioremediation of oil-contaminated lands. Environmental and Experimental Biology. 2018:105-111

[56] Abdul Khalil HPS, Saurabh CK, Tye YY, Lai TK, Easa AM, Rosamah E, et al. Seaweed based sustainable films and composites for food and pharmaceutical applications: A review. Renewable and Sustainable Energy Reviews. 2017;**77**(January):353-362

[57] Shawky HA. Improvement of water quality using alginate/montmorillonite composite beads. Journal of Applied Polymer Science. 2011;**119**(4):2371-2378

[58] Barreca S, Orecchio S, Pace A. The effect of montmorillonite clay in alginate gel beads for polychlorinated biphenyl adsorption: Isothermal and kinetic studies. Applied Clay Science. 2014;**99**:220-228

[59] Pereira L. Seaweeds as source of bioactive substances and skin care therapy—Cosmeceuticals, algotheraphy, and thalassotherapy. Cosmetics. 2018;**5**:68

[60] Malinowska P. Algae extracts as active cosmetic ingredients. Zesz Nauk/Uniwersytet Ekonomiczny w Poznaniu. 2011;**212**:123-129

[61] Fabrowska J, Łęska B, Schroeder G, Messyasz B, Pikosz M. Biomass and extracts of algae as material for cosmetics. In: Kim S, Bażyńska-Chojnacka K, editors. Marine Algae Extracts. Weinheim, Germany: Wiley-VCH Verlag GmbH & Co. KGaA; 2015. pp. 681-706

[62] Wang HMD, Chen CC, Huynh P, Chang JS. Exploring the potential of using algae in cosmetics. Bioresource Technology. 2015;**184**(December):355-362

[63] Pereira L. A review of the nutrient composition of selected edible seaweeds. In: Seaweed: Ecology, Nutrient Composition and Medicinal Uses. 2012. pp. 15-47

[64] Cervino G, Fiorillo L, Herford AS, Laino L, Troiano G, Amoroso G, et al. Alginate materials and dental impression technique: A current state of the art and application to dental practice. Marine Drugs. 2019;**19**(1):1-15

[65] Kovalenko I, Zdyrko B, Magasinski A, Hertzberg B, Milicev Z, Burtovyy R, et al. A major constituent of brown algae for use in high-capacity Li-ion batteries. Science. 2011;**334**(6052):75-79

[66] Chen H-B, Shen P, Chen M-J, Zhao H-B, Schiraldi DA. Highly efficient flame retardant polyurethane foam with alginate/clay aerogel coating. ACS Applied Materials & Interfaces. 2016;**8**(47):32557-32564

[67] Liu Z, Li Z, Zhao X, Zhang L, Li Q, Liu Z, et al. Highly efficient flame retardant hybrid composites based on

calcium alginate/nano-calcium borate. Polymers (Basel). 2018;**10**(6):625

[68] Liu Y, Zhang C-J, Zhao J-C, Guo Y, Zhu P, Wang D-Y. Bio-based barium alginate film: Preparation, flame retardancy and thermal degradation behavior. Carbohydrate Polymers. 2016;**139**:106-114

Section 2

Pharmaceutical and Medical Uses

Chapter 2

Pharmacological Effects and Utility as a Food Additive of Calcium Alginate

Fumiyoshi Kasahara, Yoko Idota, Yuuki Fukai, Chihaya Kakinuma and Takuo Ogihara

Abstract

Here we review the physiological effects of the calcium salt of alginate (Ca-Alg), focusing on our own work. First, we found that Ca-Alg promotes the excretion and decreases the absorption of various metals, and does so more effectively than sodium alginate (Na-Alg). Ca-Alg also reduced plasma cholesterol (Cho) in rats fed a high-Cho diet for 2 weeks. This was considered to be due to reduced intestinal reabsorption of bile acid, resulting from the binding of Ca-Alg and bile acid; this induces an increase of bile acid synthesis from Cho in the liver, leading to a decrease in Cho in plasma. The increase of blood triglyceride (TG) levels in rats fed a high-fat diet for 5 weeks was significantly suppressed by Ca-Alg, leading to decreased fat accumulation in the liver and whole body. Ca-Alg in food was also effective in suppressing the postprandial increase of blood glucose level in rats and humans. An in vitro study suggested that Ca-Alg inhibits the interaction between α-glucosidase and its substrate maltose. In conclusion, Ca-Alg has a number of beneficial effects as a functional food ingredient, and is expected to be a safe and effective food additive for long-term use.

Keywords: calcium alginate, toxic metal, cholesterol, bile acid, triglyceride, micelle, fat, blood glucose level, particle size, noodles

1. Introduction

Alginic acid (Alg) is a polysaccharide derived from algae. Sodium alginate (Na-Alg) is commonly used in foodstuffs as a thickening agent and stabilizer, and is also used as a health food to suppress weight gain and lower blood cholesterol (Cho) [1–4]. In addition, Na-Alg has a protective action on the gastric mucosa [5, 6]. Moreover, when Na-Alg is ingested prior to exposure to strontium (Sr), Sr accumulation in the human body is decreased [7]. However, the sodium salt of Alg can potentially cause hypertension, a major risk factor for dyslipidemia and arteriosclerosis [8]. Therefore, if the calcium salt (Ca-Alg) is as effective as, or superior to, Na-Alg, it might prove to be of greater benefit.

In this chapter, focusing on our own work on Ca-Alg, we will firstly describe how Alg enhances excretion and reduces absorption of Sr and cesium (Cs) in rats. Secondly, we discuss the relationship between the physical parameters of various metal ions and their binding affinity to Alg. Thirdly, we describe the

Cho-lowering effect of Ca-Alg, as well as the reducing effect of Ca-Alg on blood triglyceride (TG) levels, which leads to reduced accumulation of fat in the liver and whole body in rats. Finally, we describe how Ca-Alg in food (noodles) moderates the postprandial blood glucose level in rats and humans and we discuss the mechanism of this effect.

2. Increased excretion and reduced absorption of strontium and cesium

Although several years have passed since the nuclear power plant accident following a severe earthquake in Japan in March 2011, public unease over the possible presence of radioactive materials in foods remains. As we anticipated that foods or medicines containing Alg would help to reduce potential harmful effects, we investigated the effect of Alg on the absorption and excretion of Sr and Cs, whose radioactive isotopes have long half-lives (^{90}Sr 28.8 years, ^{137}Cs 30.17 years). Specifically, we examined and compared the effects of Na-Alg and Ca-Alg on the absorption and excretion of Sr and Cs in rats, as well as investigating their safety [9].

Initially, we examined the adsorption of Sr and Cs by water-soluble Na-Alg. We found that Sr alone was adsorbed by Na-Alg in a concentration-dependent manner, as was Cs alone. On the other hand, when a mixture of Sr and Cs was used, adsorption of Cs by Na-Alg was lower than in the case of Cs alone, whereas adsorption of Sr by Na-Alg was the same as with Sr alone. Thus, both Sr and Cs were concentration-dependently adsorbed by Na-Alg, but adsorption of Cs by Na-Alg was partly blocked in the presence of Sr.

Next, rats were randomized into control (normal diet), Na-Alg, and Ca-Alg groups, and the changes of native Sr and Cs concentrations in plasma were measured after 2 weeks. In the groups fed Na-Alg and Ca-Alg, the Sr concentrations were significantly decreased to 65 and 63% at 1 week, and 77 and 66% at 2 weeks, respectively, compared with the control group. On the other hand, Cs concentration was significantly reduced (to 60% of the control) only at 2 weeks in the Ca-Alg group. Histopathological observation revealed mineral deposition, due to excessive ingestion of sodium, in the pelvic epithelium of the kidney in the Na-Alg group, and epithelial hyperplasia was observed around the deposits. In contrast, no abnormality at all was detected in the Ca-Alg group. These results indicate that Ca-Alg would be safer than Na-Alg if taken daily for protection against radiation damage.

We also randomized rats into control, Na-Alg, and Ca-Alg groups, and administered $SrCl_2$ or CsCl solution. The maximum plasma concentration (C_{max}), time to C_{max} (T_{max}), and area under the concentration curve for 3 hours after administration (AUC0-3 hours) were calculated from the observed data by subtracting the values before administration. When $SrCl_2$ solution was orally administered in the Na-Alg and Ca-Alg groups, absorption of Sr was significantly decreased in comparison with the control group. In the Ca-Alg group, Cmax and AUC0–3 hours were significantly lower than in the control group after oral administration of CsCl solution. No significant difference of Cs plasma concentration profile between the control and Na-Alg groups was observed. Overall, the data suggest that absorption of both Sr and Cs was reduced in the Ca-Alg group, whereas absorption of Cs was not reduced in the Na-Alg group (**Figure 1**).

It should be noted that in these studies we used 10% Na-Alg or Ca-Alg in the diet, whereas 3–4 g/body/day of Alg is typically ingested by humans as a health food [1, 10]. Clinical studies will be required to identify an appropriate level of Ca-Alg for use as a protective agent.

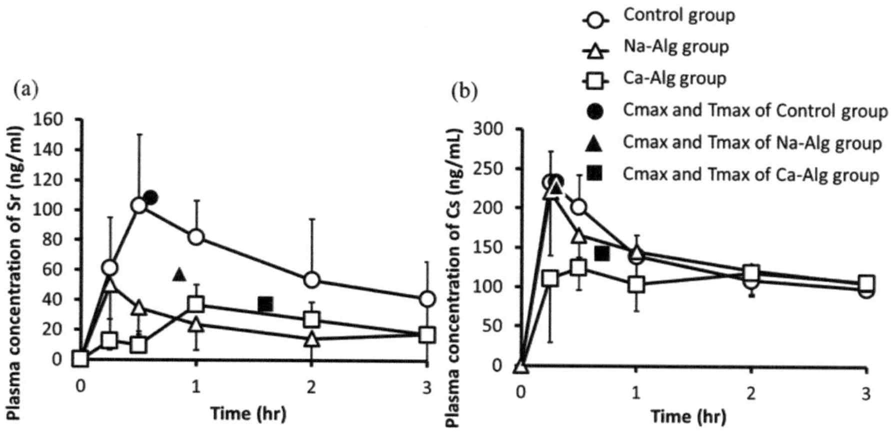

Figure 1.
Plasma concentration of Sr (a) or Cs (b) after oral administration of $SrCl_2$ to rats [9]. The data represent means ± S.D. (n = 5).

3. Mechanism of binding of alginate and metals

In the case of acute oral exposure to toxic metals, health damage can be reduced by immediate treatments such as induction of vomiting and/or the use of a laxative to promote excretion of the metal. However, in the case of chronic exposure, it is essential to use intrinsically safe absorption inhibitors and/or excretion accelerators that are suitable for long-term administration.

Although the effect of Alg on Sr or Cs absorption and excretion has already been reported, there is little information about its effect on other metals. Therefore, we investigated the relationship between the physical parameters of various metal ions, including toxic metal ions, and the binding affinity of these metal ions for Alg [11]. For this purpose, the binding constants (K, mM^{-1}) and the binding amount with Alg were evaluated for Sr, Pb, Tb, Dy, Ca, Cd, Mg, Fe(II), Fe(III), Co, Al, Ni, Cs, Cu, Ag, Li, and K. Aqueous solutions of each metal salt and an equivalent amount of Na-Alg were mixed, and the amount of unbound metal remaining in the filtrate was determined using an atomic absorption photometer. The amount of bound metal was calculated from the amount of remaining unbound metal ion, and K values and the number of binding sites per 1 mg of Alg (n) were analyzed using double-reciprocal plots. The affinity of each metal ion for Alg was calculated by multiplying the n and *K* values. Moreover, the relationships between charge number and radius of these metals and their binding affinity were examined.

The order of K values was as follows: $Sr^{2+} > Pb^{2+} > Tb^{3+} > Dy^{3+} > Ca^{2+} > Cd^{2+} > Mg^{2+} > Fe^{2+} > Fe^{3+} > Co^{2+} > Al^{3+} > Ni^{2+} > Cs^{+} > Cu^{2+} > Ag^{+} > Li^{+} > K^{+}$. Moreover, metal ions with high K values tended to have ionic radii within the range of about 90–120 pm. On the other hand, the order of affinity for Alg was $Pb^{2+} > Dy^{3+} > Tb^{3+} > Sr^{2+} > Ca^{2+} > Mg^{2+} > Cd^{2+} > Fe^{2+}, Fe^{3+} > Cs^{+} > Al^{3+} > Co^{2+} > Ni^{2+} > Cu^{2+} > Ag^{+} > K^{+} > Li^{+}$.

The *K* value and affinity for Alg both tended to be higher for divalent or trivalent metal ions than for monovalent ions. It is well established that Alg forms a cross-linked structure with divalent or trivalent metal ions, resulting in gel formation. These results might indicate that metal ions with an ionic radius of about 90–120 pm form more robust and water-insoluble gels (**Figure 2**) [11].

Overall, these results indicate that Alg would be effective as an excretion accelerator and/or absorption inhibitor for various toxic metal ions, especially divalent metals such as Pb and Cd.

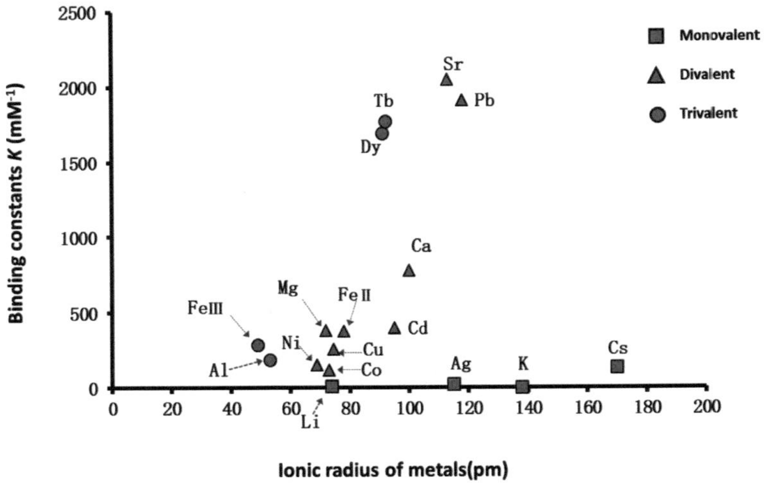

Figure 2.
Relationships between K value, charge number and ionic radius of metal ions [11].

It is noteworthy that the affinity between Alg and Cs is relatively small, even though we had previously shown that Ca-Alg is effective in promoting excretion and decreasing absorption of Cs in rats [9]. Therefore, not only the affinity between Alg and metals, but also other factors arising from the specific combination of Alg and metal ion, may influence excretion and/or absorption of individual metal ions in the presence of Alg.

4. Cholesterol-lowering effect

Heart disease and cerebrovascular disease are major causes of death in developed countries, accounting for about a quarter of all deaths in Japan [12]. A major factor in their pathogenesis is believed to be dyslipidemia [13–15], which is predominantly a modern lifestyle-related disease [16, 17]. Therefore, there is considerable interest in food additives or health foods that can decrease Cho absorption or promote Cho excretion.

Since Na-Alg reduces the Cho concentration in blood [9], we focused on the Cho-lowering effect of Ca-Alg in rats fed a high-Cho diet [18]. We first examined absorption of the Cho precursor taurocholate by various types of Alg in vitro, using Na-Alg instead of Ca-Alg, since Na-Alg is water-soluble. We found that high-molecular-weight, guluronic acid-rich (HMW-G) Na-Alg showed the greatest adsorption of taurocholate, and so we selected Ca-Alg HMW-G for the following in vivo study.

Rats were fed a high-Cho diet with or without 0.5–2% Ca-Alg for 2 weeks. After 14 days, the plasma concentration of Cho, the portal plasma concentration of bile acid, and the bile acid content in feces were measured. Moreover, in order to monitor safety, blood samples withdrawn after 14 days were used for the measurement of biochemical parameters. In the groups fed the high-Cho diet containing 2% Ca-Alg diet, the plasma concentration of Cho at 2 weeks was significantly lower than that of the group fed high-Cho diet alone. This result was similar to that in the group fed colestimide-containing diet as a positive control. Bile acid excretion in feces tended to increase depending on the concentration of Ca-Alg in the diet. In the group fed the 2% Ca-Alg diet, the portal plasma concentration of bile acid was significantly decreased, compared to that in the high-Cho diet group. Furthermore, the portal

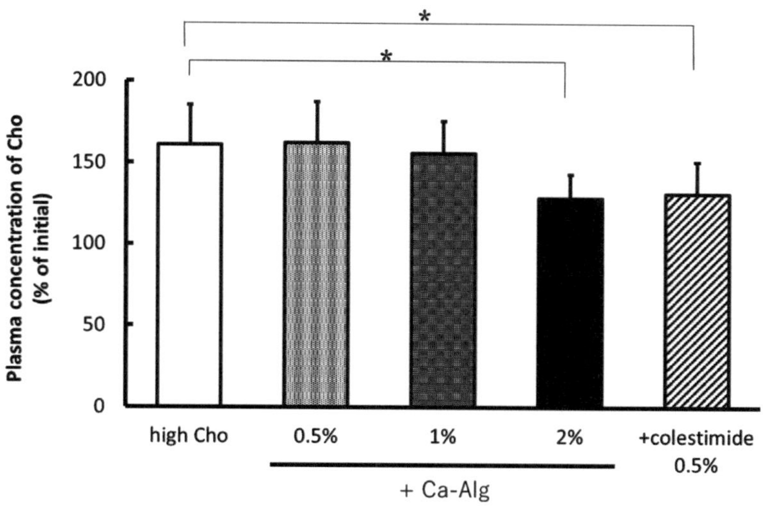

Figure 3.
Cho concentration in plasma at the end of the 2-week period with normal diet, high-Cho diet, or high-Cho diet containing Ca-Alg or colestimide to rats [18]. Rats were fed normal diet, high-cholesterol (Cho) diet, or high-cholesterol diet containing Ca-Alg or colestimide. The data represent means ± S.D. (n = 6). The significance of differences from the high-Cho diet group was determined by means of Dunnett's test. $^{*}p < 0.05$.

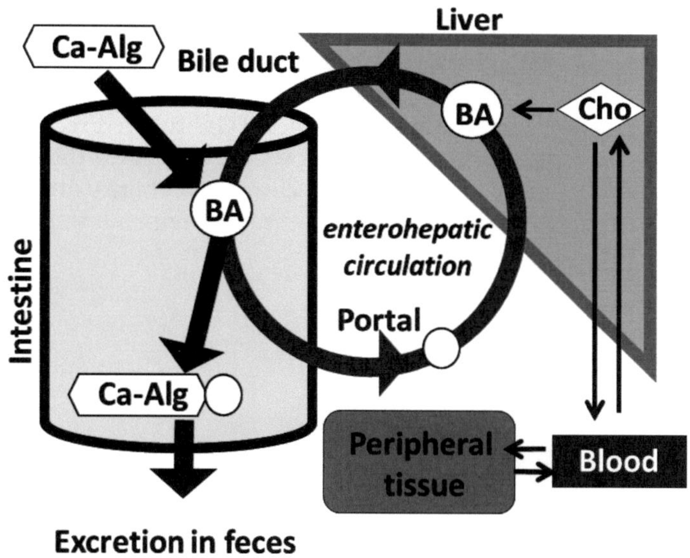

Figure 4.
A possible mechanism of Cho-lowering effect of Ca-Alg [18].

concentration of bile acid was significantly lowered in the 2% Ca-Alg group. There was no significant difference in weight gain or diet intake among the groups during the 2-week experimental period. Microvesicular steatosis was increased in the high-Cho diet and Ca-Alg groups, but remained within the physiological range. While several changes in biochemical parameters and histopathological findings were observed, all values remained within the physiological range (**Figure 3**).

Overall, these results indicate that Ca-Alg is effective for reducing plasma Cho. A possible mechanism would be enhanced fecal excretion of bile acid due to reduced intestinal reabsorption, which might subsequently stimulate bile acid synthesis from Cho in the liver, leading to a decrease of Cho in plasma (**Figure 4**).

5. Reduction of blood triglyceride levels

Excess lipid is stored in the form of TG in subcutaneous and internal organs in the body, and is broken down into fatty acids as required [19]. Dyslipidemia, with increased TG and Cho levels in the blood, leads to atherosclerosis, which in turn can lead to cardiovascular disease and stroke. Accumulation of TG can also result in fatty liver disease, leading to decreased hepatic function, liver cirrhosis and potential morbidity, including myocardial infarction, cerebral infarction and angina pectoris, and eventually cancer [20–23].

Since we previously observed that the TG level in blood was decreased by Ca-Alg in rats [18], we next set out to examine the effect of Ca-Alg on elevated TG levels in the blood, hepatic and total body accumulation of fat, and body weight in rats fed a TG-loaded diet for 5 weeks. We also investigated the mechanism of the TG-reducing effect of Alg in vitro [24].

Rats were randomized into five groups: a high-fat diet group (14% w/w lard, HF); 3 Ca-Alg-containing diet groups (2.5, 5 or 10% w/w Ca-Alg) and a resistant maltodextrin (RMD) diet group as a positive control (with 5% w/w RMD). The 10% Ca-Alg group showed a significant reduction of body weight increase from the 7th day. The increase of TG in blood was also significantly suppressed, and the amount of TG excreted in feces was increased. Increase of body fat mass was in the order HF > RMD > Ca-Alg 2.5% > Ca-Alg 5% > Ca-Alg 10%, while the total weight of the extracted fat tissues was significantly reduced in the RMD, 5 and 10% Ca-Alg groups. Hepatic pathology showed clear circular vacuoles apparently representing TG accumulation in the HF group, while fewer vacuoles were seen in the Ca-Alg groups.

These results suggest that Ca-Alg lowers blood TG through direct suppression of TG absorption, independently of its effect on Cho. As regards the mechanism of Ca-Alg action, hepatic pathology showed that clear circular fatty droplets presumed to represent TG accumulation were present in the HF group, but were reduced in

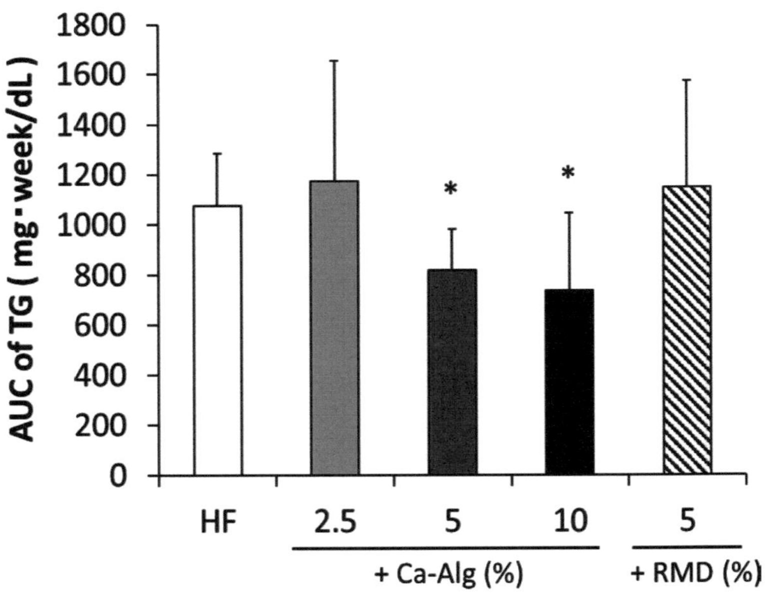

Figure 5.
*Area under the blood concentration-time curve of TG in rats after the 5-week feeding period with high-fat diet or high-fat diet containing Ca-Alg or high-fat diet containing RMD [24]. The data represent means ± S.D., n = 7. *p < 0.05, compared with high-fat diet.*

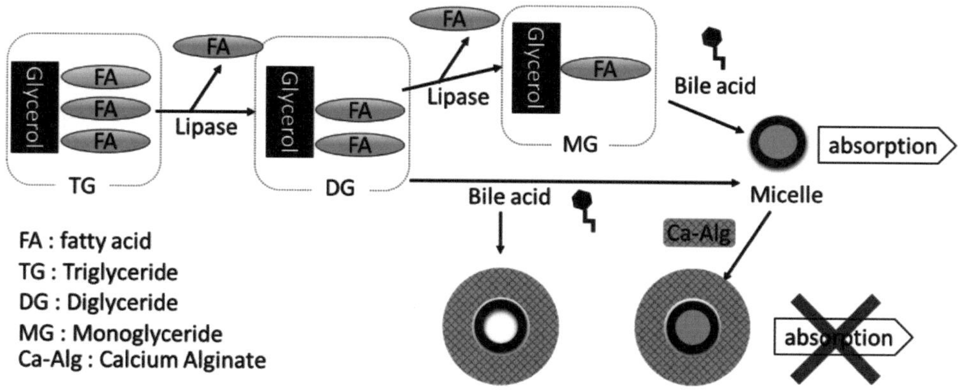

Figure 6.
A possible mechanism of TG-lowering effect of Ca-Alg [24].

the 10% Ca-Alg group. Interestingly, the concentrations of uric acid, allantoin and BUN in plasma were also decreased in all the Ca-Alg groups, though the mechanism involved is unclear (**Figure 5**).

We then investigated whether Alg affects lipase activity. Na-Alg was suspended in water, and diluted as required. When this solution was added to an emulsion composed of bile acid and lecithin in the presence of lipase, no decrease of lipase activity was observed, ruling out a direct effect on lipase. On the other hand, when Na-Alg was added to an emulsion composed of TG, bile acid and lecithin, the emulsion was well maintained, and a creaming phenomenon was confirmed after 5 days. When water was added to the emulsion, it disintegrated, precipitating lecithin and releasing TG on the liquid surface. These results suggest that Alg stabilizes bile acid micelles containing TG, possibly by absorbing them and forming large micelles that cannot be absorbed, or that are less vulnerable to lipases [24].

These results suggest that Ca-Alg suppresses absorption of TG, leading to reduced blood TG levels, and decreases hepatic and total body accumulation of TG, in addition to promoting excretion. These findings should help to provide a rational basis for designing future clinical trials (**Figure 6**).

6. Suppression of postprandial blood glucose level

Diabetics may develop serious complications such as retinopathy, nephropathy and neuropathy, in addition to myocardial infarction, cerebral infarction and so on [27, 30], even though the initial subjective symptoms may be minor. Ca-Alg is known to suppress the postprandial increase of blood glucose, and therefore may be helpful in preventing lifestyle-related diseases such as diabetes. Starch is initially decomposed to maltose in the gastrointestinal tract, mainly by α-amylase, before decomposition by α-glucosidase (maltase) to glucose. Transporters located on the cell membrane surface absorb glucose. Ca-Alg should inhibit at least one of these processes to suppress blood glucose levels since it is not absorbed from the gastrointestinal tract. We therefore chose to investigate which of these processes is inhibited by Ca-Alg, and the optimal amount and particle size of Ca-Alg in the diet required to suppress the postprandial increase of blood glucose in rats [25].

We first examined the effect of Ca-Alg concentration on α-glucosidase activity, and observed no significant change compared to the control. On the other hand, the amount of glucose adsorbed on Ca-Alg increased with increasing initial glucose concentration until it reached saturation. The direct binding affinity of glucose for

Ca-Alg was low, and the values of the permeation coefficient of glucose showed no significant change. Moreover, it has been reported that the addition of Alg (polysaccharides) increases the viscosity of starch suspension, and there is a positive correlation between apparent viscosity and the decrease of starch digestion [26]. We speculate that Ca-Alg interferes physically with contact between α-glucosidase and maltose by increasing the viscosity of the intestinal contents. It was our assumption that blood glucose suppression by Ca-Alg is the result of decreased efficiency in starch digestion due to the inhibition of α-glucosidase. This may be as a result of increased viscosity of the gastrointestinal contents. We next aimed to define the optimum amount and particle size of Ca-Alg in the diet for the suppression of postprandial blood glucose levels in rats [25]. A diet containing starch together with varying amounts and particle sizes of Ca-Alg was orally administered to rats randomized into five groups: starch with no Ca-Alg (control), or with Ca-Alg (3%; 270 mesh pass, 5%; 270 mesh pass, 5%; 150 mesh pass, or 5%; 80 mesh pass) (n = 3–4 each). Blood was sampled and the glucose level was measured before administration (C_0). Water was added to the five types of starch with or without Ca-Alg and the mixtures were orally administered to conscious rats. Blood glucose levels were measured and the change in blood glucose level (ΔC_n) was calculated. Starch containing 5% Ca-Alg (particle size; 270 mesh pass) significantly decreased the ΔC_{max} and ΔAUC, compared to starch containing no Ca-Alg. However, 3% 270-mesh-pass Ca-Alg, or 5% 150- or 80-mesh-pass Ca-Alg produced no significant difference in ΔC_{max} or ΔAUC compared with the 0% Ca-Alg diet (**Figure** 7) [25].

The in vivo study determined 5% of 270-mesh-pass Ca-Alg to be the most efficient combination of amount and particle size in the suppression of postprandial increases in blood glucose. Compared with 0% Ca-Alg, significant decreases were observed in both ΔC_{max} and ΔAUC, confirming a decrease in both postprandial peak glucose level and the full amount of glucose absorbed within 2 hours of ingestion. It seems likely that the magnitude of action would depend on the surface area of Alg.

Our results support the idea that Ca-Alg increases the viscosity of the gastrointestinal contents, depending upon the surface area of the administered gel. The gel is expected to interfere with the interaction between α-glucosidase and maltose, thereby suppressing the production of glucose, and preventing a sharp rise in blood glucose level. Various products have been reported to moderate glucose absorption; for example, indigestible dextrin has been confirmed to suppress the postprandial increase in blood glucose level by inhibiting α-glucosidase activity [28]. It seems

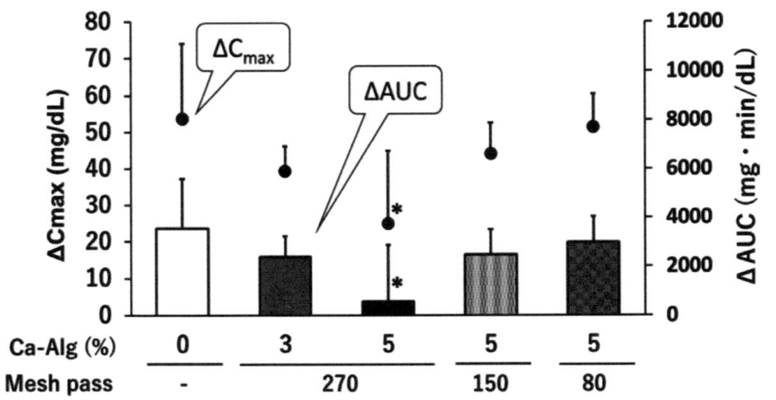

Figure 7.
*Effect of starch diets containing Ca-Alg on blood glucose level in rats [25]. Circles: ΔC_{max}, the difference between the maximum blood glucose level C_{max} and the pre-feeding blood glucose level C_0. Bars: ΔAUC, the difference between the area under the blood glucose level-time curve from 0 to 120 min after ingestion and the baseline value C_0. The data represent means ± S.D., n = 3 or 4. *p < 0.05, compared with control.*

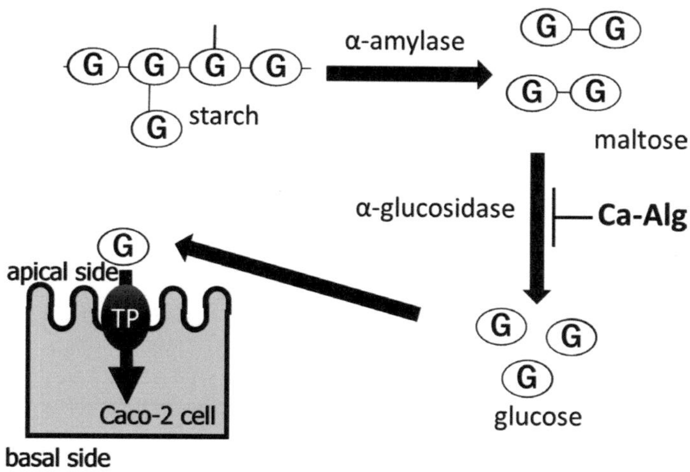

Figure 8.
A possible mechanism of blood glucose level-lowering effect of Ca-Alg [25].

reasonable to consider that Ca-Alg works similarly. Moreover, it was found that 5% of 270-mesh-pass Ca-Alg was the most effective combination of amount and particle size to suppress the postprandial increase of blood glucose (**Figure 8**).

To analyze the effect of Ca-Alg on the postprandial increase of blood glucose, a prospective, randomized, double-blind, 3-group, 3-phase crossover study was undertaken among healthy Japanese adult subjects [29]. Traditional Japanese udon noodles were selected, and blood glucose levels were measured after ingestion of Ca-Alg-free udon, and noodles containing 5 or 8% Ca-Alg. We also examined the effect of Ca-Alg on other chemical parameters in plasma or serum. Healthy male and female volunteers of 20 years of age or older were divided into three groups so that the average BMI values in the groups were similar. Each group ingested one of the three types of noodles containing 0 (control), 5 or 8% Ca-Alg (weight % to flour and modified starch). Blood was collected by fingertip puncture for blood glucose measurement prior to feeding and after ingestion. The blood glucose level was measured twice at each point using a simple blood glucose meter, and the average value was calculated. After eating the noodles, subjects were given a tasting questionnaire to evaluate "chewiness", "thickness" and "favorability" of the noodles in a 5-point grading system (**Figure 9**).

Noodles containing 5 or 8% Ca-Alg caused a significant decrease in ΔC_{max} compared to control noodles. Moreover, ΔAUC also showed a significant decrease in both groups. No significant difference in the time of maximum blood glucose level (T_{max}) was observed among the three groups. This is consistent with previous findings [31] and is similar to findings with α-glucosidase inhibitors, [32, 33] except miglitol [34]. These results indicate that Ca-Alg suppresses the postprandial increase in blood glucose and reduces the total absorption amount of glucose, but without delaying the absorption. Thus, our previous finding that 5% Ca-Alg had a blood glucose-suppressing effect in rats [25] was reproduced in humans.

As for blood biochemical parameters, no significant difference in the amount of Ca change at 30 min after noodle feeding (ΔCa30min) was found between the 5 and 8% Ca-Alg groups compared to the control, but ΔCa at 120 min (ΔCa120 min) showed a significant increase in both groups. In addition, ΔT-Cho30 min showed a slight tendency to decrease in both groups, and ΔT-Cho120 min was slightly decreased in the 8% Ca-Alg group. There was no significant change in other blood test values. We found that the blood Ca concentration at 120 min after eating 5 or 8% Ca-Alg-containing noodles remained within the normal range, 8.5–10.4 mg/dL, [35]

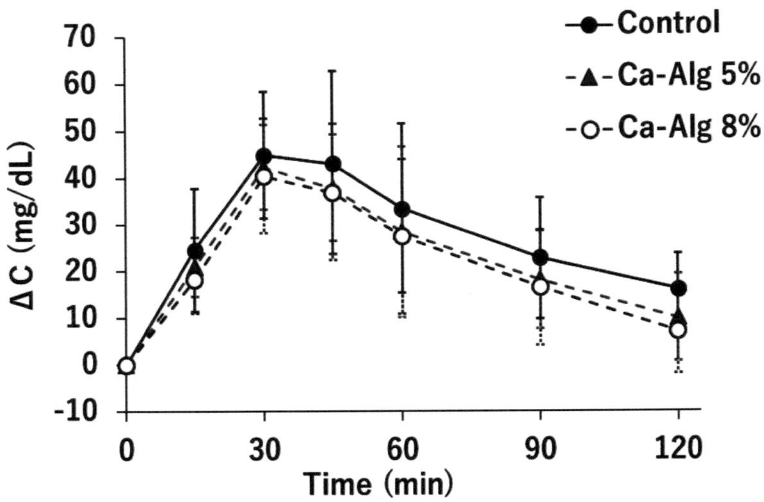

Figure 9.
Changes in blood glucose level (ΔC) after eating test noodles to volunteers [30]. The data represent means ± S.D., n = 15.

but was significantly increased compared with the value in the control noodle group, suggesting that Ca derived from Ca-Alg was absorbed into the body.

The recommended amount of Ca intake in adults to help prevent diseases such as osteoporosis is 600–900 mg/day.[35] Since the amounts of Ca in noodles containing 8% Ca-Alg and 5% Ca-Alg would be 500 and 320 mg, respectively, about half of the recommended daily intake might be provided by these noodles. The upper limit of tolerable daily Ca intake for Japanese adults is 2500 mg, [35] so even if these noodles were eaten three times a day, the upper limit would not be reached. Thus, the likelihood of excessive Ca intake appears to be low.

Many substances are known to suppress glucose absorption; for example, indigestible dextrin has been shown to inhibit α-glucosidase. Our work showed that Ca-Alg also inhibits α-glucosidase activity [25], and its effect on blood glucose level was similar to or more potent than that of indigestible dextrin [36]. On the other hand, α-glucosidase inhibitors have side effects such as abdominal distention and flatus. Ingestion of noodles containing 8% Ca-Alg was expected to show an α-glucosidase-inhibitory effect equal to about 1/40th that of a single dose of acarbose [21]. Therefore, it is considered that the likelihood of side effects arising from α-glucosidase inhibition due to ingestion of noodles containing Ca-Alg is extremely low.

Our results raise the interesting possibility that the introduction of food ingredients containing Ca-Alg into the regular diet may be helpful in preventing lifestyle-related diseases, particularly diabetes and osteoporosis, without adversely affecting individual eating habits.

7. Conclusion

Alg, especially Ca-Alg, has a number of beneficial physiological effects. For example, we have shown that Ca-Alg increases excretion and reduces the absorption of toxic heavy metals such as Sr. and Cs in rats. Moreover, Ca-Alg decreases the blood Cho and TG levels, as well as reducing plasma levels of uric acid, allantoin and BUN levels in rats. Further, Ca-Alg moderated the postprandial increase of blood glucose level in rats and humans. Ca-Alg has been confirmed as safe for use as a food additive, and is superior to Na-Alg, because there is no risk of hypertension

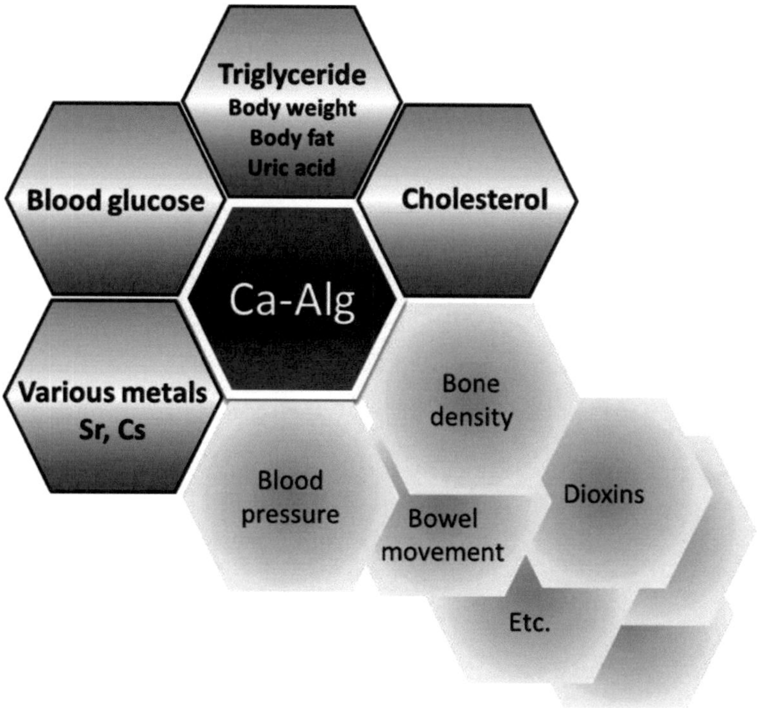

Figure 10.
Revealed functions and future development of Ca-Alg.

due to increased sodium intake. In addition, Ca-Alg may also have a preventive effect on osteoporosis. Ca-Alg is convenient to take, because it is effective in solid form, and it appears to be suitable for long-term use as an additive or functional food (**Figure 10**).

Lifestyle-related diseases associated with high calorie intake and insufficient exercise have become a significant social problem [37, 38], and may lead to the development of cancer, heart disease and cerebrovascular disease, which are major causes of death [13–17, 23, 39, 40]. It will be interesting to examine further whether Ca-Alg may also offer potential benefits in relation to lifestyle-related diseases [36].

Acknowledgements

This work was supported by JSPS Grant-in-Aid for Challenging Exploratory Research (KAKENHI) Grant Number 25560062.

Conflict of interest

Fumiyoshi Kasahara is an employee of Kimica Corporation. The other authors have no potential conflicts of interest.

Author details

Fumiyoshi Kasahara[1,2], Yoko Idota[1], Yuuki Fukai[1], Chihaya Kakinuma[1] and Takuo Ogihara[1*]

1 Faculty of Pharmacy, Takasaki University of Health and Welfare, Takasaki-shi, Gunma, Japan

2 Kimica Corporation, Tokyo, Japan

*Address all correspondence to: togihara@takasaki-u.ac.jp

References

[1] Kimica Corporation Web. 2019. Available from: https://kimica-algin.com/alginate/about/ [Accessed: 23 April 2019]

[2] Nishizawa M, Kuda T, Yamagishi T, Tsuji K. Effect of depolymerized sodium alginate on the excretion of cholesterol from rats. Journal Home Economic Japan. 1997;**48**:689-693. DOI: 10.11428/jhej1987.48.689

[3] Peters HP, Koppert RJ, Boers HM, Ström A, Melnikov SM, Haddeman E, et al. Dose-dependent suppression of hunger by a specific alginate in a low-viscosity drink formulation. Obesity (Silver Spring). 2011;**19**:1171-1176. DOI: 10.1038/oby.2011.63

[4] Georg Jensen M, Kristensen M, Astrup A. Effect of alginate supplementation on weight loss in obese subjects completing a 12-week energy-restricted diet: A randomized controlled trial. The American Journal of Clinical Nutrition. 2012;**96**:5-13. DOI: 10.3945/ajcn.111.025312

[5] Pharmaceuticals and Medical Devices Agency Web. 2013. Available from: http://www.info.pmda.go.jp/downfiles/ph/PDF/200343_2329116S1094_2_01.pdf [Accessed: 23 April 2019]

[6] Asaoka T, Iwatuka H, Minowa H. Effect of "CHOLECUT", a drink containing depolymerized sodium alginate, on serum total cholesterol levels in healthy males. Japanese Journal of Nutritional Assessment. 1996;**13**:460-464

[7] Hesp R, Ramsbottom B. Effect of sodium alginate in inhibiting uptake of radiostrontium by the human body. Nature. 1965;**208**:1341-1342

[8] Fujita T, Henry WL, Bartter FC, Lake CR, Delea CS. Factors influencing blood pressure in salt-sensitive patients with hypertension. American Journal of Medicine. 1980;**69**:334-344. DOI: 10.1016/0002-9343(80)90002-9

[9] Idota Y, Harada H, Tomono T, Morimoto K, Kobayashi S, Kakinuma C, et al. Alginate enhances excretion and reduces absorption of strontium and cesium in rats. Biological & Pharmaceutical Bulletin. 2013;**36**: 485-491. DOI: 10.1248/bpb.b12-00899

[10] Hayashi H, Ohno S, Arai T, Suzuki N. Examination of several FOSHU used in hypercholesterolemia. Japanese Journal Complementary and Alternative Medicine. 2008;**5**:183-196. DOI: 10.1625/jcam.5.183

[11] Idota Y, Kogure Y, Kato T, Yano K, Arakawa H, Miyajima C, et al. Relationship between physical parameters of various metal ions and binding affinity for alginate. Biological & Pharmaceutical Bulletin. 2016;**39**:1893-1896. DOI: 10.1248/bpb.b16-00127

[12] Trends in Leading Causes of Death, Summary of Vital Statistics. Ministry of Health, Labour and Welfare. 2015. Available from: http://www.mhlw.go.jp/english/database/db-hw/populate/dl/03.pdf [Accessed: 23 April 2019]

[13] Kitamura A, Iso H, Naito Y, Iida M, Konishi M, Folsom AR, et al. High-density lipoprotein cholesterol and premature coronary heart disease in urban Japanese men. Circulation. 1994;**89**:2533-2539. DOI: 10.1161/01.CIR.89.6.2533

[14] Iso H, Naito Y, Sato S, Kitamura A, Okamura T, Sankai T, et al. Serum triglycerides and risk of coronary heart disease among Japanese men and women. American Journal of Epidemiology. 2001;**153**:490-499. DOI: 10.1093/aje/153.5.490

[15] Lida M, Ueda K, Okayama A, Kodama K, Sawai K, Shibata S, et al. Impact of elevated blood pressure on mortality from all causes, cardiovascular diseases, heart disease and stroke among Japanese: 14 year follow-up of randomly selected population from Japanese (Nippon Data80). Journal of Human Hypertension. 2003;**17**:851-857. DOI: 10.1038/sj.jhh.1001602

[16] Teramoto T. Dietary management in Japan atherosclerosis society (JAS) guidelines for the prevention of atherosclerotic cardiovascular diseases in Japanese—2012 version. The Japanese Journal of Nutrition and Dietetics. 2013;**71**:3-13. DOI: 10.5264/eiyogakuzashi.71.3

[17] Abifadel M, Varret M, Rabès JP, Allard D, Ouguerram K, Devillers M, et al. Mutations in PCSK9 cause autosomal dominant hypercholesterolemia. Nature Genetics. 2003;**34**:154-156. DOI: 10.1038/ng1161

[18] Idota Y, Kogure Y, Kato T, Ogawa M, Kobayashi S, Kakinuma C, et al. Cholesterol-lowering effect of calcium alginate in rats. Biological & Pharmaceutical Bulletin. 2016;**39**:62-67. DOI: 10.1248/bpb.b15-00503

[19] Shibata S, Ikeda Y. Chrono-nutrition of macro-nutrition including lipids. Journal Lipid Nutrition. 2015;**24**:53-60. DOI: 10.4010/jln.24.53

[20] Koda M, Kawakami M, Murawaki Y, Senda M. The impact of visceral fat in nonalcoholic fatty liver disease:Cross-sectional and longitudinal studies. Journal of Gastroenterology. 2007;**42**:897-903. DOI: 10.1007/s00535-007-2107-z

[21] Vega GL, Chandalia M, Szczepaniak LS, Gruda SM. Metabolic correlates of nonalcoholic fatty liver in women and men. Hepatology. 2007;**46**:716-722. DOI: 10.1002/hep.21727

[22] Jakobsen MU, Berentzen T, Sorensen TI, Overvad K. Abdominal obesity and fatty liver. Epidemiologic Reviews. 2007;**29**:77-87. DOI: 10.1093/epirev/mxm002

[23] Eguchi Y, Eguchi T, Mizuta T, Ide Y, Yasutake T, Iwakiri R, et al. Visceral fat accumulation and insulin resistance are important factors in nonalcoholic fatty liver disease. Journal of Gastroenterology. 2006;**41**:462-469. DOI: 10.1007/s00535-006-1790-5

[24] Kasahara F, Kato T, Idota Y, Takahashi H, Kakinuma C, Yano K, et al. Reduction effect of calcium alginate on blood triglyceride levels causing the inhibition of hepatic and total body accumulation of fat in rats. Biological & Pharmaceutical Bulletin. 2019;**42**:365-372. DOI: 10.1248/bpb.b18-00530

[25] Tajima N, Noda M, Origasa H, Noto H, Yabe D, Fujitda Y, et al. The Japan Diabetes Society: Evidence-based practice guideline for the treatment for diabetes in Japan 2013. Diabetology International. 2015;**6**:151-187. DOI: 10.1007/s13340-015-0206-2

[26] Kopf D, Frölich L. Risk of incident Alzheimer's disease in diabetic patients: A systematic review of prospective trials. Journal of Alzheimer's Disease. 2009;**16**:677-685. DOI: 10.3233/JAD-2009-1011

[27] Idota Y, Kato T, Shiragami K, Koike M, Yokoyama A, Takahashi H, et al. Mechanism of suppression of blood glucose level by calcium alginate in rats. Biological & Pharmaceutical Bulletin. 2018;**41**:1362-1366. DOI: 10.1248/bpb.b18-00155

[28] Sasaki T, Kohyama K. Influence of non-starch polysaccharides on the in vitro digestibility and viscosity of starch suspensions. Food Chemistry. 2012;**133**:1420-1426. DOI: 10.1016/j.foodchem.2012.02.029

[29] Tashiro M, Kato M. Effect of administration of indigestible dextrin prepared from corn starch on glucose tolerance in streptozotocin-diabetic rats. Journal of Japan Society of Nutrition and Food Science. 1999;**52**:21-29. DOI: 10.4327/jsnfs.52.21

[30] Kato T, Idota Y, Shiragami K, Koike M, Nishibori F, Tomokane M, et al. Randomized, double-blind, crossover clinical trial of the effect of calcium alginate in noodles on postprandial blood glucose level. Biological & Pharmaceutical Bulletin. 2018;**41**:1367-1371. DOI: 10.1248/bpb.b18-00156

[31] Sawabe A, Fukuda Y, Ueno M, Kawachi Y, Takeda R, Komemushi S. Effect of postcibal blood triglyceride level and blood glucose level by single intake of calcium alginate content food for adult men. Dietary Research. 2013;**33**:41-46

[32] Glucobay (Acarbose) tablet interview form. 2019. Available from: http://www.info.pmda.go.jp/go/interview/1/630004_3969003F1026_1_001_1F.pdf [Accessed: 23 April 2019]

[33] Basen (Voglibose) tablet interview form. 2017. Available from: https://www.med.takeda-teva.com/di-net/product/doc/1/06/1106_BASEN_tab_ODtab_IF.pdf [Accessed: 23 April 2019]

[34] Seibule (Miglitol) tablet interview form. 2017. Available from: http://med.skk-net.com/supplies/products/item/SBL_if_1706.pdf [Accessed: 23 April 2019]

[35] Ministry of Health, Labour and Welfare. Dietary reference intakes for Japanese. 2015. Available from: www.mhlw.go.jp/file/05-Shingikai-10901000-Kenkoukyoku-Soumuka/0000114399.pdf [Accessed: 23 April 2019]

[36] Kishinaga Y, Yamada F, Nambu S. Effects of the coffee containing resistant maltodextrin on postprandial blood glucose level—A randomized double-blind crossover study. Japanese Pharmacology and Therapeutics. 2014;**42**:347-351

[37] WHO. Global Status Report on Non-Communicable Diseases 2014. Geneva: World Health Organization; 2014. Available from: http://www.who.int/nmh/publications/ncd-status-report-2014/en/ [Accessed: 2019 April 23]

[38] Watanabe T. Food and disease: The etiological background of so-called lifestyle-related diseases. Journal of Japan Society of Nutrition and Food Science. 2004;**57**:15-19. DOI: 10.4327/jsnfs.57.15

[39] Ministry of Health, Labour and Welfare. 2016: Analysis by Cause of Death. Available from: http://www.mhlw.go.jp/english/database/db-hw/lifetb16/dl/lifetb16-04.pdf [Accessed: 23 April 2019]

[40] Stamler J, Rose G, Stamler R, Elliott P, Dyer A, Marmot M. INTERSALT study findings. Public health and medical care implications. Hypertension. 1989;**14**:570-577. DOI: 10.1161/01.HYP.14.5.570

Chapter 3

Current Perspective and Advancements of Alginate-Based Transplantation Technologies

Samuel Rodriguez, Rahul Tuli, Ashlyn Wheeler, Amy Nguyen, Jennifer Luong, Reza Mohammadi, Michael Alexander and Jonathan R.T. Lakey

Abstract

Versatile yet biocompatible bio-materials are in high demand in nearly every industry, with biological and biomedical engineering relying heavily on common biomaterials like alginate polymers. Alginate is a very common substance found in various marine plants which can easily be extracted and purified through cheap nonhazardous methods. A key characteristic of alginate polymers includes easily manipulatable physical properties due to its inert but functional chemical composition. Factors including its functional versatility, long-term polymer stability and biocompatibility have caused alginate-based technologies to draw major attention from both the scientific and industrial communities alike. While also used in food industry manufacturing and standard dental procedures, this chapter will focus on a discussion of the both clinical and nonclinical use of alginate-based technologies in transplantation for regenerative cell and drug delivery systems. In addition, we overview the immune system response prompted following implantation of alginate hydrogels. Consequences of immune cell reactivity to foreign materials, such as inflammation and the foreign body response (FBR), are also analyzed and current and future strategies for potential circumvention of severe immune responses toward alginate-based devices are reviewed and suggested.

Keywords: alginate, biomaterial, foreign body response, inflammation, transplantation, pancreatic islet, stem cell, microencapsulation

1. Introduction

Alginate was first described in the 1880s by the British chemist E.C.C Stanford after extracting it from seaweed using a rudimentary ion exchange method [1]. After the commencement of commercial production in the late 1920s, alginate became a widely used substance in several industries due to it numerous useful and nontoxic attributes. By the middle of the twentieth century, alginate was a major contributor to the food industry as a food-stabilizer. Today, Alginate-derived products contribute to the seaweed industry which had an annual production value of over $4.1 billion USD in 2017 [2].

2. Sources of alginate

2.1 Brown algae source

Contributing up to 40% of the dry matter, a major raw source of alginic acid is derived from marine algae and kelp-like brown seaweed [3, 4]. There are several species of brown algae from which alginate can be derived; however, two species, namely *Macrocystis porifera* and *Ascophyllum nodosum*, account for most of the world's supply of alginate [5]. These species of seaweed are members of a class of seaweed that are both large and lengthy, making these plants ideal for alginic acid harvesting [5]. Unlike eukaryotic animal cells, plant cells are known to contain a rigid cell wall composed mainly of carbohydrate polysaccharide like cellulose and pectin [6]. Marine plants, such as algae, contain cell walls which are maintained by hydrocolloid polysaccharides such as alginate, carrageen, and agar which differentiate aquatic vegetation from land plants [6, 7]. These precursors can be used to cultivate alginic acid for market production.

2.2 Bacterial exopolysaccharide alginate source

Two types of gram-negative bacteria genera, namely *Pseudomonas* and *Azotobacter*, can produce alginate in the form of exopolysaccharides which constitute bacterial biofilm [8, 9]. For example, *Pseudomonas aeruginosa* can synthesize alginate which contributes to the mucosal buildup of biofilms along the respiratory tract of patients with the disease cystic fibrosis [10–12]. The biosynthesis of alginate in these bacteria genera are conducted through genetic expression of alginate substrate producing genes (alg), the products of which are exported to the cell exterior [9]. The isolation of marginally pure alginate from immobilized bacterial cell extracts has been reported, but the progress of advanced bacterial alginate isolation techniques has been slow overall [13, 14]. Although these bacteria can be utilized as a source of alginate, the main commercially available form of alginate is derived from brown algae sources.

2.3 Alginate extraction

Alginate exists *in vivo* as a mixture of different alginate salts including magnesium, strontium, or calcium within the intracellular matrix of brown algae tissue [4, 15]. Alginate is the conjugate base of the alginic acid and is formed upon treatment with alkaline medium [4, 16]. The primary extraction of alginic acids from brown seaweed is performed using an alkaline ion exchange treatment method which can extract and separate each of the major carbohydrate constituents of the brown algae [8, 17]. The initial extraction of algal particles from brown algae results in semi-pure fractions of differing polysaccharides which include the salt form of alginate [18, 19]. A chemical purification process, usually $CaCl_2$ purification, involves treatment of algal particles with a mineral acid followed by neutralization with strong base (**Figure 1**). Alginate precipitates are formed via further ion transfer acid-base reaction which results in a product of mainly sodium alginate [4, 8, 18]. The sodium alginate form of alginic acid is the most favored form produced after extraction which is mainly due to cold water solubility [16]. Current techniques examine the quality and purity of extracted alginate during extraction and purification processes through several chemistry-based analytical assays including nuclear magnetic resonance (NMR) and infrared (IR) spectroscopy [16, 20]. Recent advances in computational modeling have allowed

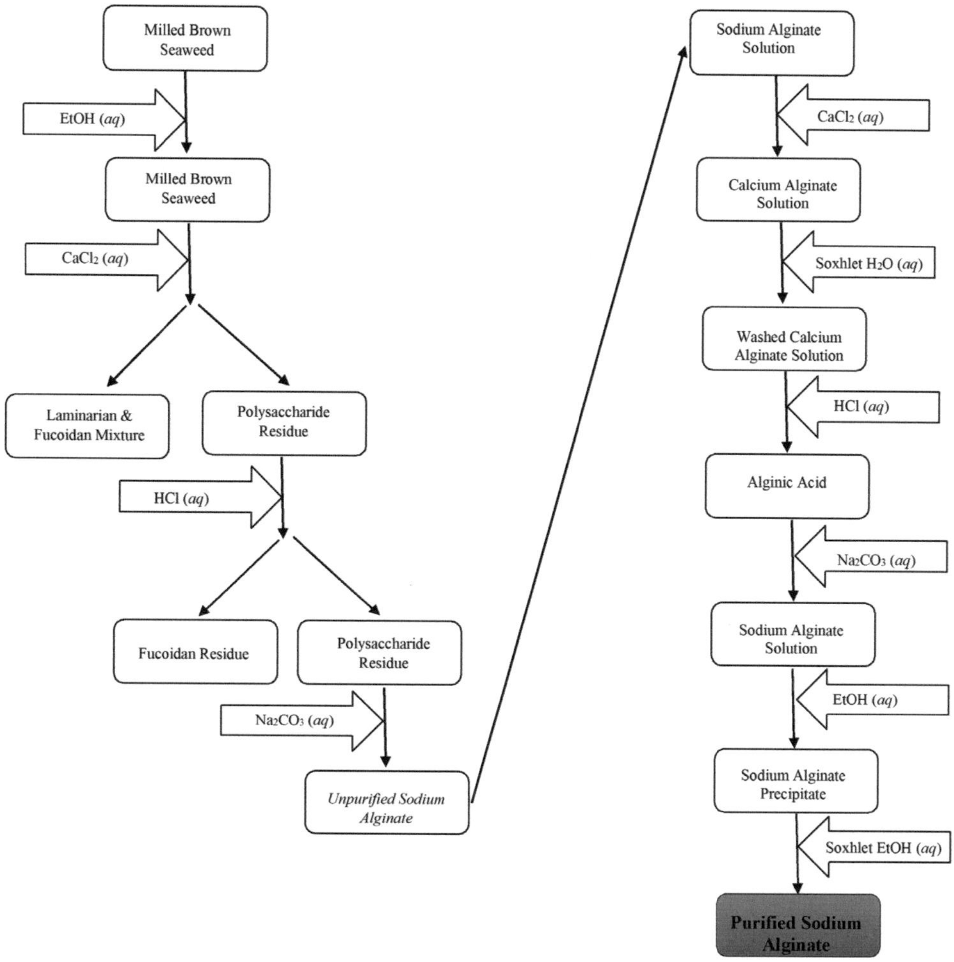

Figure 1.
Extraction of sodium alginate from brown seaweed followed by sodium alginate purification via $CaCl_2$ purification.

researchers to construct models of precipitation stages which has allowed for optimization of the extraction and purification process overall [20].

3. Composition of alginate

3.1 Types of alginate polymers

Alginate is an unbranched copolymer of β-D-mannuronic acid (M group) and α-L-guluronic acid (G group) commercially derived from algae [8]. Hydroxyl and carboxyl groups are abundantly distributed across the polymer, giving rise to a plethora of chemically modifiable sites [21]. Commercially, alginate is blocked in either consecutive M, consecutive G, or alternating M & G [22]. Given that it is a polymer with versatile properties, alginate can be easily changed to exhibit a variety of properties tailored to the individual needs of an implant. Pre-existing properties of alginate are able to be chemically enhanced through manipulating the percentage of M and G in the material, adding immunoprotective layers that impede diffusion, as well as divalent cation crosslinking. Under dicationic conditions, viscous alginate transforms into a gel, which can then be used as an encapsulation medium for islet cells [23–25]. M groups lie with the main ring in an equatorial conformation, with each mer connected covalently through an ether (**Figure 2**). With dications situating on top and on bottom of each layer, a "swelling" effect is noted as there is no discrete pocket between mers resulting in each linear polymer stacking on top of the crosslinking dication. In contrast, G groups lie with the main ring axial (**Figure 3**). These mers are also attached through an ether. However, these ethers create pockets large enough for dications to situate without creating a swollen stacking effect. Manipulation of molecular weight and composition (%G or %M) leads to varying strength and porosity of the gel [26, 27]. Generally, alginates with higher %G have higher comparative levels of elasticity and stability [22].

Along with *Macrocystis porifera* and *Ascophyllum nodosum*, another type of brown seaweed that is a main source of alginate is called *Sargassum polycystum* C. Agardh. One study extracted alginate from *S. polycystum* to examine its chemical makeup and viscosity in the leaf, stem and thallus regions [28]. Thallus of seaweed refers to undifferentiated tissues where nutrient uptake and gas exchange occurs [29]. Of the structures studied for *S. polycystum*, the leaf region was found to have the highest alginate yield followed by the stem region and the thallus [28]. In contrast, the viscosity of alginate was highest in the stem region, followed by the leaf region and thallus [28]. Of the M/G ratios observed, the stem region had the lowest M/G ratio and the highest level of G-block content, optimal properties of forming a rigid and stable gel [28]. Similarly, other commercial brown seaweeds such as the stems of *Laminaria hyperborea* have a high G-block content (70%) and a low M/G ratio (0.43) [30].

3.2 UPLVM

Purified alginate containing almost entirely M blocks with little to no G blocks will typically not yield the ideal type of hydrogel desired through dication crosslinking. The lack of pockets available for crosslinking will result in a form of layers of alternating alginate polymers and dications. In terms of structural integrity, UPLVM alginate will be less porous and strong, allowing higher malleability. In addition, although there has been no clear consensus, studies have suggested that a greater percentage of M blocks in alginate cause an increased immune response compared to UPLVG alginate, as indicated by increased production of TNF-α, IL-1 and IL-6 [31].

3.3 UPLVG

Alginate with a higher %G blocks (>60% G) will result in a material a higher polymer strength and available crosslinking sites for barium atoms [27]. Since there are sites for divalent cation network crosslinking, the cations will situate themselves in the "egg carton" that the G blocks form. The cations in this position

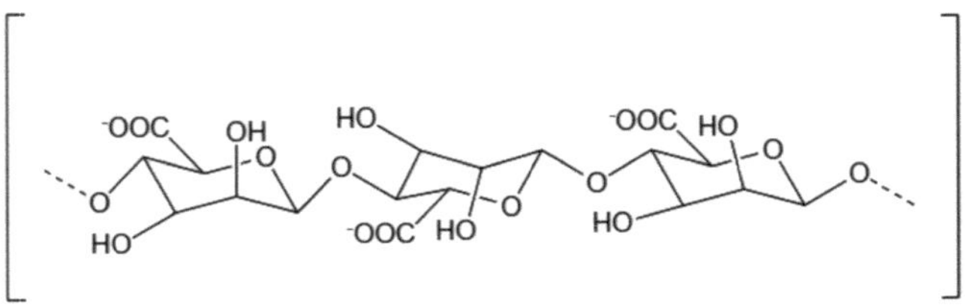

Figure 2.
Chemical structure of M-block monomer.

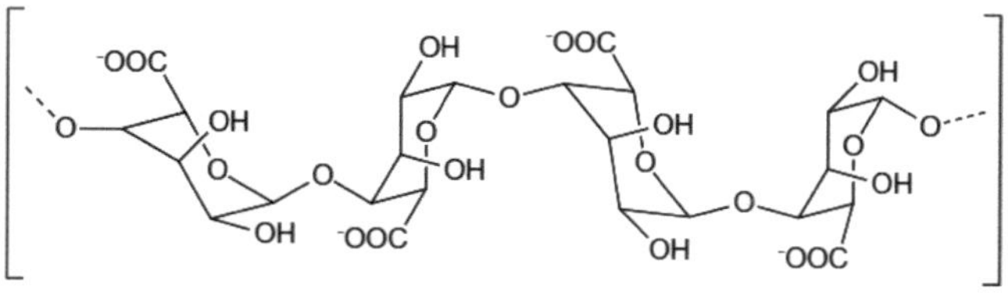

Figure 3.
Chemical structure of G-block monomer.

create a resistance to shear and frictional forces that the layers undergo as alternating molecular weight increases [32]. Therefore, this orientation allows for higher density, strength and porosity. The carboxylate anions that lie equatorial in G blocks are usually protonated under acidic conditions, which are deprotonated as the basicity of the solution increases [33]. The alcohol groups also present in the polymer provide a hydrogen that is capable of being deprotonated in basic conditions. Although this pH change resistance results in an increased stability of G-rich polymers against depolymerization, pH changes in solution will result in swelling of alginate capsules [34].

3.4 Mixtures

Alginate is commercially sold as a mixture of M & G blocks with varying purification. NovaMatrix in Norway is a widely used company that manufactures and distributes purified alginates [34]. Their UP LVG (ultrapure low viscosity, high G) alginate has at least a 1.5:1 ratio of G:M blocks, with UP LVM (ultrapure low viscosity, high M) alginate having a ratio of G:M of less than 1. NovaMatrix recommends a shelf life of 5 years for their UP LVG alginate while only 3 years for UP LVM alginate. Both types of alginate should ideally be stored in a fridge and maintained at a relatively neutral pH (between 5 and 8) so as to decrease the rate of depolymerization. Higher temperatures will result in an increased rate of polymerization, which is expanded even further in the presence of an acid or a base. A neutral pH will prevent acid or base catalysts from recruiting oxygen to initiate oxidative-reductive depolymerization. Both M-rich and G-rich alginates react with no significant difference when base catalyzed, but M-rich alginates are hypothesized to be more vulnerable to acid catalyzed depolymerization, as supported by a catalytic constant that is twice as large for M-rich alginates than that of G-rich alginates [35]. In addition, in the presence of oxygen and an acidic or alkaline environment, the phenol and carboxylate groups will react in undesired ways, resulting in free radical depolymerization.

3.5 Alginate derivatives

Alginate derivatives have also been created to encompass certain properties. One example of this is amphiphilic alginate derivatives that utilize the alginate backbone and synthesize it with hydrophobic moieties [8, 36]. An example of this is sodium alginate being conjugated with long alkyl chains via ester bonds [36]. The microparticles for the derivative are prepared using dispersion in a sodium chloride solution; this allows for encapsulation of proteins and their subsequent release by adding surfactants to disrupt intermolecular hydrophobic junctions or esterases that hydrolyze the ester bond between the alginate backbone and alkyl chains [36]. Other types of derivatives include dodecylamine conjugated to an alginate backbone via amide linkage which leads to long-term stability in aqueous media compared to other alginate derivatives composed of dodecyl esters which have a risk of hydrolysis [36]. Amphiphilic alginate derivatives that are water soluble have also been developed using cholesteryl groups which are synthesized using N,N′-dicyclohexylcarbodiimide as a coupling agent and 4-(N,N′-dimethylamino) pyridine as a catalyst at room temperature [37]. Other derivatives include cell-interactive alginates which are composed of cell-adhesive peptides. To prepare these, carbodiimide chemistry is used to combine peptide side-chains with carboxylic groups on sugar molecules [36]. This is important because alginate must acquire the proper ligands to participate in cell-to-cell interactions since it does not innately have cell-adhesivity to mammalian cells [36]. The peptide sequence arginine-glycine-aspartic acid (RGD) has been studied widely due to the copious integrin receptors for this ligand on a variety of cell types [38]. This, among other types of cell-interactive alginates, has been used for scaffolds for tissue engineering and 2-D and 3-D cell culture matrices.

4. Current biotechnological uses

4.1 Food industry applications

The alginate industry saw increases in production in response to the scientific advancements in the study of alginate properties and potential uses [39]. Currently, the FDA classifies alginate as meeting the guidelines of the Food Chemical Codex and lists over seven different uses of it in the food industry [40]. The primary market for alginate in the processed food market where they serve as texturing agents and food stabilizers [41]. The gel-like chemical properties, which are safe for consumption, also allow for several other uses such as increasing storage life of potatoes, immobilization of banana enzymes, immobilization of lactic acid bacteria, and fillers in meat and fish products [39, 42]. The ability of alginate hydrogel to be polymerized, or gelled, into a microcapsule with a hollow core has led to the development of food encapsulation technologies aimed at food preservation [42]. Recently, researchers have shown that application of an alginate coating on egg shells has led to the elimination of cross-contamination from *Salmonella enteritidis* for up to 42 days [43]. Currently in the beverage industry, alginate is used as an emulsifying agent to maintain the stability of foam within beverages like beer [44, 45]. Continued use in the food industry will likely increase the commercial demand of alginate in the future.

4.2 Pancreatic islet cell-delivery system

In 1933, Biscegeli implanted polymer matrix coated murine-derived tumor cells in to the abdomen of guinea pigs which remained viable without rejection, thus discovery prompted entire fields to research into microencapsulation technologies [46]. Several advances in biotechnological approaches to both cell microencapsulation and the development of drug delivery systems using alginate have been achieved for nearly 50 years [47]. When reconstituted in aqueous solution, alginate forms a hydrogel which in the presence of polyvalent cation (e.g., Ba^{2+}, Ca^{2+}, Sr^{2+}) reorganizes into a rigid biomaterial [4]. Alginate hydrogels can be used to encapsulate cellular tissue and nonliving substances for therapeutic cellular-delivery as a treatment to many diseases such as Type 1 Diabetes [48]. Xenograft transplantations for type 1 diabetes heavily rely on alginate hydrogels as a source biomaterial for encapsulation of porcine pancreatic islets. Key obstacles observed with porcine islet xenograft include possible transmission of hemagglutinating and lymphocytotoxic antigens, such as carbohydrate α-(1,3)-galactose, which are a major contributor to acute host immune rejection [49–51]. Alginate encapsulation, in contrast to other biomaterials, reduces transmission of humoral immune response elements while allowing for the transport of nutrients and export of insulin across the semipermeable barrier [52]. Recently, alginate-encapsulated APIs were transplanted intraperitoneally into STZ-induced IDDM nonhuman primates. Nonhuman primates exhibited a marked decrease in exogenous insulin demands and lower %HbA1C in addition to normalized blood glucose values for 20–70 days. However, the glycemic control was reduced over time, which they concluded was due to decreased graft function and viability [53].

4.3 Stem cell-delivery system

With the application of FDA regulations and recent advances in stem cell-related technologies, there has been an increase in need for viable targeted delivery system for therapeutics [54–57]. The biocompatibility and relative ease of production of alginate hydrogels makes alginate an important candidate for production of immune-isolated stem cell delivery systems [8, 58, 59]. A major disease model currently researching stem cell-related therapies is for the treatment of type 1 diabetes, among insulin-dependent conditions. Recently, insulin-producing human SC-derived β-cells encapsulated with alginate polymers were implanted in immune-competent mice. Multiple studies report glycemic control with immuno-isolated β-cells in mice, some resulting in up to 174 days of glycemic correction, in addition to detection of human C-peptide in mouse serum [60, 61]. A 2019 study showed similar results after transplanting human pluripotent stem cell-derived (iPSCs) β-cells into immunocompetent mice which resulted in glycemic control for more than 150 days [62]. Other disease models have also used alginate microencapsulation for therapeutic use of xenogeneic stem cell-delivery. Researchers have reported functional alginate encapsulated adrenal SCs for use in adrenal hormone insufficiency diseases [63, 64]. Successful alginate encapsulation of neural embryonic stem cells was also reported for targeted cell-delivery serving possible treatment for neural tissue repair in several neurological disorders [65]. Microencapsulation of stem cells is a very active field of research and advances with this technology have a wide range of clinical applications.

4.4 Cryoprotective use of alginate microencapsulation

Transplantations can sometimes rely heavily on transportation or storage of tissues before the procedure. Cryopreservation, known as a viable option for tissue preservation and storage, can have severe effects on the viability and function of tissues during the freezing/thawing processes and from use of cryoprotective agents [66]. Alginate microcapsules have demonstrated the ability to maintain structure, slow cooling process, reduce effects of ice crystal formation on tissue, and regulate influx of cryoprotective agents during cryopreservation [67, 68]. First used in preservation of plant cells, use of an alginate coating has been observed to have cryoprotective properties [69–72]. Success with plant cell preservation catalyzed the research into alginate cryoprotective potential with other tissue types. Alginate coatings of beneficial probiotic bacteria have demonstrated maintenance of viability and function through the cryopreservation process which has potential applications in yogurt and probiotic preservation [73–75]. An augmented necessity of tissue preservation methods has caused a rise in research related to cryopreservation for storage and distribution of animal cells. Alginate microencapsulation of cells offers significant degree of cryoprotection during cryo processing [76, 77]. Transplantation research has particularly benefited from use of alginate technologies during cryopreservation. Recent studies in pancreatic islet transplantation have demonstrated that use of alginate microencapsulation helps maintain islet viability during preservation and improves islet secretory function during transplantation [67, 78, 79]. A 10 years study using encapsulated rat, pig, human islets showed that alginate encapsulated islets maintained significantly higher viability, secretory function, and yield compared to nonencapsulated islets after cryopreservation for 10 years [80]. Like pancreatic islets grafts, cryopreservation is also used for preservation of stem cells before transplantation. Alginate encapsulation has been shown repeatedly to improve both yield and function of multiple stem cell lines, including human stem cells [81, 82]. Recently, the use of alginate microcapsules improved viable recovery of human adipose-derived stem-cells after 72-h storage in hypothermic conditions [83]. The overall benefits of cryoprotection via alginate encapsulation will ensure relevance in future research of cell preservation and transplantation.

4.5 Conjugated alginate potential as drug-delivery system

Due to the relative feasibility of conjugation and semi-permeable wall structure of alginate microcapsules shows promising secretory capabilities for robust nanoparticle drug-delivery systems [8, 84–86]. Recently researchers have been able to conjugate alginate microcapsules with anti-HIV zidovudine nanoparticles. Results showed significant improvements in internalization of the nanoparticle into glioma cells during *in vitro* experiments marking for potential use as a targeted viral drug delivery system [87]. Another study demonstrated the conjugation of sodium alginate with graphene oxide which is known to create functional groups for synthesis. GO-conjugated alginate hydrogels readily loaded the anticancer drug oxorubicin hydrochloride (DOX·HCl) and caused high cytotoxicity when exposed to immortal HeLa cell lines [88]. When islet containing alginate microcapsules were conjugated with VEGF, increases in angiogenesis, islet viability, and islet function were observed [89]. More recently, similar benefits were observed through increases in bone formation and blood vessel growth after biomineral-conjugated alginate microcapsules containing MSCs were transplanted into sheep with ovine iliac crest bone defects [90]. The versatile conjugation behavior of alginate hydrogels has impressive potential for a variety of future medical applications in transplantation.

5. Immune response

5.1 Alginate purity effect on immunogenicity

Crude unpurified alginate has been shown to provoke the immune system which then causes fibrosis around the microcapsule [91]. This overgrowth of immune-cells and fibroblasts interferes with the transfer of nutrients, hormones, and other proteins via the semi-permeable membrane of the capsule [92]. This is a difficult problem to avoid especially since the industrial processing used for extraction can leave contaminates in the alginate like polyphenols, endotoxins and algal proteins [92, 93]. Purification is a technique utilized to minimize the amount of contaminations in the alginate gels. Commercially available sodium alginate can be purchased in several different purified states including "ultra-purified" form from companies like Novamatrix® for use in hydrogel production [94–96]. Although this is highly purified there are still small concentrations of contaminants in the alginate that can prompt a severe foreign body response [91, 97]. If the alginate biomaterials hold living tissue within a drug-delivery system, the foreign body reaction tends to reduce the survivability of those tissues [92, 98].

5.2 Inflammation and the foreign body response

The human immune system is broken into two parts, the innate and adaptive immune systems, which both work in tandem to defend and destroy external bacteria, viruses and various other microbes that may infiltrate a host's body [99]. The first aspect of the foreign body response (FBR) is the innate immune system which has no flexibility or memory to foreign antigens. This is followed by the adaptive immune system which generates a custom response to each specific pathogen while simultaneously building an immunological memory [92]. Alginate hydrogels used in implantations are highly purified so as to not present antigens on their surface and thus should not cause T cell activation due to antigen-presentation [100]. Despite lacking these immunoreactive properties, within nanoseconds of entering a host, biomaterials initiate an inflammatory FBR due to biomaterial surface interactions with tissue, proteins, and blood [100, 101]. The foreign body response results in fibrotic overgrowth surrounding the implanted alginate hydrogels which essentially isolates the biomaterial from host's body [102]. This fibrotic overgrowth is initiated by a sequence of cascading events including injury formation, recruitment of immune cells and fibroblasts, and cell adhesion which leads to fibrous tissue deposition [103]. Two stages of inflammation, namely acute followed by chronic, facilitate the foreign body response once alginate biomaterials are implanted [102].

It was determined that the immunogenic properties of alginate polymers were not directly responsible for the overgrowth around capsules but do contribute to is formation. In order for the immune cells to adhere to the cell surface, there must be a significant amount of protein adsorption or anchor sites for immune cell adhesion [92, 102]. Instead, the immune response occurs in the tissue immediately surrounding the alginate structure [92]. Studies have demonstrated that within a few days after alginate biomaterial implantation into animals, immune cells and differentially activated macrophages (i.e., stadia, granulocytes, and basophils) collect around, but not on, the alginate surface [92, 104]. This acute inflammatory period is characterized by the recruitment of macrophages and neutrophils in addition to the release of histamine and fibrinogen adsorption from mast cells to surrounding tissue [92, 102]. This is all done without significant immune cell adhesion to alginate biomaterials. A key player in immune cell recruitment are pattern recognizing receptors (PRRs) which act as sensors on cells of the innate immune system by responding to evolutionary conserved molecules with can contaminate alginate biomaterials [92]. Even after purification, lipoteichoic acid and LPS, the most commonly known endotoxin, can remain and are recognized by Toll-like Receptors (TLRs) [52]. It has been demonstrated that recognition of PAMPs by TLRs causes the activation of macrophages through the NF-κB pathway [105]. NF-κB results in the transcriptional upregulation of genes most associated with cytokine and chemokine production which serve to intensify humoral response [105]. Within a week, the initial acute inflammatory period transitions to a chronic inflammatory period.

The chronic inflammatory stage is characterized by the accumulation of lymphocytes and monocytes, among other mononuclear cells, in the tissue surrounding the alginate biomaterial [106, 107]. It was discovered *in vitro* that lymphocytes can adhere to alginate biomaterial surfaces, but when placed in co-cultures with macrophages, they appeared to attach predominantly to the macrophage rather than the alginate microcapsule surface [100]. Further research has suggested that macrophage adhesion and fusion to biomaterial surface is assisted by T lymphocytes [100]. Both macrophages and lymphocytes secrete inflammatory mediators. Examples of these include cytokines IL-1β, IL-6, and TNFα and chemokines IL-8, MCP, MIP-1β, and ENA-78, all of which are known to activate and recruit inflammatory effector cells such as neutrophils, monocytes, T lymphocytes, and natural killer cells [100, 105]. Similarly, it was discovered that certain cytokine, chemokine levels, matrix metalloproteinases (MMPs) and tissue inhibitor MMPs (TIMP), fluctuated over time which suggests that T lymphocyte-macrophage interactions have the ability to facilitate the chronic inflammatory phase of the FBR [100, 108]. There have been *in vivo* studies that have shown active T cells in response to synthetic materials during an inflammatory response; however, *in vitro* studies have shown a lack of lymphocyte response to alginate biomaterials [100, 109]. A novel focus of study regarding mitogens, which are functional groups on the surface of biomaterials, led to the hypothesis that they can possibly trigger lymphocytes via cross-linking of glycoproteins, but these mitogenic properties have not been observed [100]. The chronic inflammatory period usually subsides 2 weeks after implantation and any longer periods of inflammation are usually the result of infection [100, 102]. A combination of granulation, fibroblast infiltration, and macrophage/fibroblast surface adhesion result in the final fibrotic encapsulation of alginate biomaterials.

5.3 Immuno-modulation of alginate hydrogels

To overcome the challenges of inflammation and fibrosis associated with the foreign body response after alginate hydrogels are implanted, researchers are currently trying to establish technologies for potential immune modulation. Research into alginate immune-modulation methods currently involves the use of bioactive nanoparticles, immune regulatory cells, hydrogel surface topography, and passive non-fouling agents [110]. In the past bioactive nanoparticles, like ketoprofen, have shown potential to modulate the degree of inflammation during FBR [111]. A recent study was able to load monoclonal antibody IgM nanoparticles during alginate encapsulation of pancreatic islets. This resulted in localized controlled release of the monoclonal antibody after implantation which decreased the immune response against transplants [112]. An islet transplantation study using the anti-inflammatory nanoparticle rapamycin, demonstrated reduced fibrosis and sustained glycemic control improvement [113]. Mesenchymal-derived stem cells have been shown to have a wide range of regenerative effects on several tissue injury types because of their multipotent capacity [114]. Several recent studies have demonstrated immune modulation of alginate hydrogels through co-delivery of MSCs with cell-delivery systems. This can help reduces inflammation and can modulate T-cell toxicity while also boosting wound healing properties and blood vessel formation of the graft site [115–117]. A better understanding of the mechanism of FBR in the future will help improve immune modulation technologies for transplantations involving alginate hydrogels.

6. Clinical relevance of alginate-based biomaterials

6.1 Type 1 diabetes mellitus treatment

While extensively performed in animal models for several decades, islet xenotransplantations have taken more time in advancing to clinical human studies around the world. This is because the area of xenografts in general is still a highly regulated area in the transplantation field and is being studied heavily in animal models [118, 119]. In the United States, the stringent FDA regulations for all xenotransplantations has provided certain standards which must be achieved pre-clinically before moving to clinical trials [120]. This has made initiation of clinical trials involving alginate xenografts very slow in the United States. Nonetheless, here have recently been a small amount of clinical islet xenotransplantation trials that have been conducted outside of the US using porcine islet xenografts to treat IDDM in human subjects (**Table 1**). The first phase I/IIa clinical trial saw 7 T1DM patients receive up to 3 implantations of encapsulated neonatal porcine islets which resulted in 5 patients with improved blood glucose levels and two patients which achieved insulin independence for up to 32 weeks post-transplantation [121, 122]. From 2000 to 2003 in a clinical trial in Mexico, two cohorts totaling 21 IDDM patients underwent xenograft implantation of a collagen-covered pre-vascularized scaffold which housed 250,000 islets with 30,000–100,000 Sertoli cells. After the first transplantation HbA1C showed significant reductions, with decreases in exogenous insulin demands observed for up to 4 years, and glucose stimulated C-peptide detected in urine for up to 4 years; in addition, zoonotic transmission of porcine microorganisms was not detected for the duration of the study [123–125]. Unfortunately, the human clinical trial in Mexico did not include a control population under exogenous insulin therapy that could further validate the results [121]. In patients who received a steroid-based regimen 33–62% decrease in insulin requirements for up to 1 year with detectable presence of porcine C-peptide compared to two patients, which received steroid-free regimen, who saw change in IDDM conditions [126]. A comprehensive 2011 study, 14 IDDM patients were given 5000–20,000 IE/kg intraperitoneally via laparoscopy using wild-type pre-weaned juvenile porcine islets without immunosuppressive therapy for 52 weeks [127]. Overall, 8 of the 14 patients showed a moderate decrease in insulin administration and HbA1C levels. A nonsignificant reduction in severe hypoglycemic events, or unaware hypoglycemic episodes, was also observed in the same patients [127, 128]. Alginate-based macrodevices have been the topic of heavy research since the late 1940s and recently have been tested clinically as a scaffold for therapeutic islet-delivery [115]. Patients with T1D have been subcutaneously implanted with macroencapsulated, bioartificial pancreatic βAir (BetaO2 Technologies Ltd., Israel) device; the study designed to monitor for 180 days post-transplantation followed by removal of the device, and 6 months of follow-up afterwards. The device involved oxygen pumps which allowed for daily refueling of oxygen to devices while in-vivo. For the duration of the study, islets in the device did not face any immune rejection and survived to time of explant. Although there were no rejections in the body, the overall efficacy of the islets was low and metabolic control was absent; C-peptide levels were detected on day 1 of post-transplantation in all patients (range 0.028–0.093 nmol/L) and remained detectable up until 2–4 weeks but for one patient detectable up to 3 months post-transplantation [129, 130]. Continued research into alginate immune-isolation of pancreatic islet xenografts will continue to develop and will be tested clinically in the future.

6.2 Wound healing treatment

Alginate has shown effectiveness as a constituent of acellular matrix skin grafts to reduce wound healing duration, which is especially poor with diabetic patients

Number of subjects (n)	Porcine islet types used	Number of islets transplanted/ kg of body weight	Transplantation site	Study outcome	Reference
12	Neonatal + Sertoli cells encapsulated in scaffold	14,000–21,000	Scaffold in subcutaneous space	• Deceased exog-enous insulin requirement for up to 4 years (50%) • No serum C-peptide detected	[124, 125]
7	Encapsulated neonatal	5000–1000	Intraperitoneal space	• Two patients achieve independence for 32 weeks • 6 Patients demonstrate lower HBA1c	[154]
1	Encapsulated fetal	15,000	Intraperitoneal space	• -12-week period of 30% reduction in insulin requirement • Improvement in glycemic control for 14 weeks • Detectable C-peptide for 11 months • Live Islet detected for 9.5 years	[127]
14	Encapsulated pre-weaned	5000–20,000	Intraperitoneal space	• Moderate decrease in insulin requirement in 57% of patients • Major reduction in hypoglycemic episodes	[127]
8	Encapsulated pre-weaned	5000–20,000	Intraperitoneal space	Patients that received 20,000/kg maintain 7% HbA1c for 600 days. Reduced Hypoglycemic events	[123]

Table 1.
Selected clinical encapsulated islet xenotransplantations in humans. IE is used to denote islet equivalents that make up the graft which are implanted during transplantation.

[131–133]. A large multicenter study involving 75 patients with 100 wounds (50% UT grade 3 wounds) was conducted using an alginate containing GraftJacket® matrix skin graft. The study resulted in 91% of complete wound closure averaging around 9.6 weeks indicating the graft was a safe option for complex lower extremity wounds [134]. Recent clinical studies with an alginate containing skin graft known as AlloPatch® have shown the effectiveness in wound healing even when elevated HbA1C levels witnessed in one patient [135]. Several alginate-based skin grafts are commercially available for advanced wound healing which include Nu-Gel® (Systagenix), Tegagel® (3M GmbH)), Curasorb® Alginate (Medtronic), Sorbsan® (B. Braun Melsungen AG), and Kendall™ Hydrocolloid Dressing (Medtronic) [136]. Advances in the development of alginate matrices will continue to contribute to skin regeneration therapy improvements in the future.

6.3 Clinical uses in dentistry

The hydrophilic nature of alginate along with hydrogel forming and biocompatible nature has made it a staple hydrocolloid for application in the field of dentistry [137]. Alginate-based gels have traditionally been used in dentistry to provide the dentist with impressions of teeth and bitemarks which can then be used as a template for dental implants [138–140]. Alginate is frequently used in clinical trials to obtain impressions when comparing various dental procedures [141–144]. In a recent clinical trial, silicone was found to be favored among patients in terms of comfortability although alginate impressions were found to be a cheaper procedure option [145, 146]. Alginate-containing matrices have also been tested for advanced periodontitis treatment, when compared to the normal 0.2% chlorhexidine treatment alginate-containing Emdogain® saw significant reduction in plaque viability [147]. These alginate-containing enamel matrices have also shown significant clinical regenerative capabilities for periodontal disease symptoms such as intrabony defects and gingival recession [148, 149].

7. Future direction for alginate-based biotechnologies

The development and use of alginate macro/micro devices for implantation have met both improvements and challenges. Specifically, alginate has been used in the production of microcapsules as well as scaffolds as a way to implant encapsulated islet cells in *vivo*. The use of natural polymers such as alginate introduces immunogenic and foreign body responses, which impact the functionality of the device over time [150]. For example, the mechanical integrity or structure of the device could be compromised, or it can decompose while inside the recipient. As a potential solution, alginate can be chemically modified so its properties can be better controlled against inflammatory response and mechanical stress [151]. This chemical modification includes both ionic and covalent crosslinks within alginate polymers which will increase the mechanical stability of both scaffolds and microcapsules [151]. This method of using two types of crosslinking to create the microbeads compared to using only covalent crosslinking has shown results of greater stability of these microcapsules within cells after weeks following implantation [151]. Furthermore, in the long run, purification techniques of alginate hydrogels can be improved to decrease PAMP concentration which would help reduce FBR [92]. Purifying alginate gels of PAMPs can be difficult for those with a high G content, which are stronger and more viscous. However, the use of chemical extraction or dialysis methods as well as specific purification methods would be required to remove these molecules. Another potential solution to overcome graft failure is to use smaller islet cell graft volumes with vascularized membranes to produce stable neovascularization near the grafted tissue [152]. Using a macroencapsulation device such as TheraCyte and loading it with islet cells of smaller volume can increase blood supply near the site of encapsulation [152].

Given the molecular composition of alginate and its ability to crosslink and form hydrogels, this biomaterial can be used in an array of medical and clinical applications. Unfortunately, the implantation of alginate induces an immune response of the host, producing setbacks that current labs are attempting to solve. Because of both macrophages mediated and T-cell mediated immune response, the alginate macro/micro device loses its viability and long-term function once it is implanted in the host. Strategies aiming to reduce or prevent fibrosis on alginate encapsulated cells present conflicting results. Newly developed capsules contain alginate without a polycation layer shown improvement potential because the pro-inflammatory characteristic of polycations have been connected to fibrotic growth around capsules [153]. For alginate beads, removing the polycation layer can lead to less stability and more permeability to cytokines and growth factors [153].

Currently, the main focus regarding implantable alginate hydrogels is to address problems such as immune response, adequate sources of oxygen, and fibrosis. As more alginate-based devices are being brought into clinical application, these strategies among others should be considered and pursued for current and future alginate-based device production.

Acknowledgements

A special thank you to the Department of Surgery at UC Irvine Medical Center and University of California, Irvine along with the Brownstein Family Trust for generous support and donations.

Conflict of interest

The authors declare that there is no "conflict of interest" with respect to this review.

Author details

Samuel Rodriguez[1], Rahul Tuli[1], Ashlyn Wheeler[1], Amy Nguyen[1], Jennifer Luong[1], Reza Mohammadi[1], Michael Alexander[1] and Jonathan R.T. Lakey[1,2*]

1 Department of Surgery, University of California Irvine, Orange, CA, USA

2 Department of Biomedical Engineering, University of California Irvine, Irvine, CA, USA

*Address all correspondence to: jlakey@uci.edu

References

[1] Stanford EC. On Algin, A new substance obtained from some of the commoner species of marine algae. American Journal of Pharmacy (1835-1907). 1883;**1**:617. DOI: https://search.proquest.com/docview/89680091?accountid=14509

[2] Dawande R. Seaweed market by product (red, brown, and green) and application (human food, hydrocolloids, fertilizers, animal feed additives, and others) - Global Opportunity Analysis and Industry Forecast, 2018-2024. Allied Market Research: 2018. p. 231

[3] Khotimchenko YS, Kovalev VV, Savchenko OV, Ziganshina OA. Physical-chemical properties, physiological activity, and usage of alginates, the polysaccharides of brown algae. Russian Journal of Marine Biology. 2001;**27**(1):S53-S64. DOI: 10.1023/A:1013851022276

[4] Draget KI, Smidsrød O, Skjåk-Broek G. Polysaccharides and Polyamides in The Food Industry: Properties, Production, and Patents. Hoboken: Wiley; 2005. pp. 1-30. DOI: https://www.cabdirect.org/cabdirect/abstract/20053218153

[5] McNeely WH, Pettitt DJ. Algin. In: Whistler RL, BeMiller JN, editors. Industrial Gums: Polysaccharides and their Derivatives. 2nd ed. New York: Academic; 1973. pp. 1-50. DOI: https://www.bcin.ca/bcin/detail.app?id=135861

[6] Rutledge RD, Wright DW. Biomineralization: Peptide-mediated synthesis of materials. In: Scott R, editor. Encyclopedia of Inorganic Chemistry. Hoboken: Wiley; 2009:1-24. DOI: 10.1002/0470862106.ia355

[7] Percival E. The polysaccharides of green, red and brown seaweeds: Their basic structure, biosynthesis and function. British Phycological Journal. 1979;**14**(2):103-117. DOI: 10.1080/00071617900650121

[8] Pawar SN, Edgar KJ. Alginate derivatization: A review of chemistry, properties and applications. Biomaterials. 2012;**33**(11):3279-3305. DOI: 10.1016/j.biomaterials.2012.01.007

[9] Remminghorst U, Rehm BH. Bacterial alginates: From biosynthesis to applications. Biotechnology Letters. 2006;**28**(21):1701-1712. DOI: 10.1007/s10529-006-9156-x

[10] Ramsey DM, Wozniak DJ. Understanding the control of *Pseudomonas aeruginosa* alginate synthesis and the prospects for management of chronic infections in cystic fibrosis. Molecular Microbiology. 2005;**56**(2):309-322. DOI: 10.1111/j.1365-2958.2005.04552.x

[11] Gacesa P, Russell NJ. The structure and property of alginate. In: Pseudomonas Infection and Alginates. London: Chapman & Hall; 1990. pp. 29-49. DOI: 10.1007/978-94-009-1836-8_3

[12] Nivens DE, Ohman DE, Williams J, Franklin MJ. Role of alginate and its O acetylation in formation of *Pseudomonas aeruginosa* microcolonies and biofilms. Journal of Bacteriology. 2001;**183**(3):1047-1057. DOI: 10.1128/JB.183.3.1047-1057.2001

[13] Richard A, Margaritis A. Empirical modeling of batch fermentation kinetics for poly(glutamic acid) production and other microbial biopolymers. Biotechnology and Bioengineering. 2004;**87**(4):501-515. DOI: 10.1002/bit.20156

[14] Lebrun L, Junter GA, Jouenne T, Mignot L. Exopolysaccharide production by free and immobilized microbial cultures. Enzyme

and Microbial Technology. 1994;**16**(12):1048-1054. DOI: 10.1016/0141-0229(94)90141-4

[15] McHugh DJ. A Guide to the Seaweed Industry, FAO Fisheries Technical Paper 441. Food and Agriculture 941 Organization of the United Nations, 2003. Available at: http://www.sidalc.net/cgi-bin/wxis.exe/?IsisScript=FAONI.xis&method=post&formato=2 &cantidad=1&expresion=mfn=000376

[16] Fertah M, Belfkira A, Taourirte M, Brouillette F. Extraction and characterization of sodium alginate from Moroccan *Laminaria digitata* brown seaweed. Arabian Journal of Chemistry. 2017;**10**:S3707-S3714. DOI: 10.1016/j.arabjc.2014.05.003

[17] Calumpong HP, Maypa AP, Magbanua M. Population and alginate yield and quality assessment of four Sargassum species in Negros Island, Central Philippines. Hydrobiologia. 1999;**398**:211-215. DOI: 10.1023/A:1017015824822

[18] Gomez CG, Lambrecht MV, Lozano JE, Rinaudo M, Villar MA. Influence of the extraction–purification conditions on final properties of alginates obtained from brown algae (*Macrocystis pyrifera*). International Journal of Biological Macromolecules. 2009;**44**(4):365-371. DOI: 10.1016/j.carres.2007.05.022

[19] Mian AJ, Percival E. Carbohydrates of the brown seaweeds *himanthalia lorea, bifurcaria bifurcata*, and *Padina pavonia*: Part I. extraction and fractionation. Carbohydrate Research. 1973;**26**(1):133-146. DOI: 10.1016/S0008-6215(00)85030-2

[20] Mohammed A, Bissoon R, Bajnath E, Mohammed K, Lee T, Bissram M, et al. Multistage extraction and purification of waste *Sargassum natans* to produce sodium alginate: An optimization approach. Carbohydrate Polymers. 2018;**198**:109-118. DOI: 10.1016/j.carbpol.2018.06.067

[21] He W, Xie Y, Yang J. Research progress on chemical modification of alginate: A review. Carbohydrate Polymers. 2011;**84**:33-39. DOI: 10.1016/j.carbpol.2010.11.048

[22] Andersen T et al. 3D cell culture in alginate hydrogens. Microarrays (Basel, Switzerland), MDPI. 2015

[23] Van der Linden E, Paques J, van Rijn CJM, Sagis L. Preparation methods of alginate nanoparticles. Advances in Colloid and Interface Science. 2014;**209**:163-171. DOI: 10.1016/j.cis.2014.03.009

[24] Thu B, Bruheim P, Espevik T, Smidsrød O, Soon-Shiong P, Skjåk-Bræk G. Alginate polycation microcapsules: I. Interaction between alginate and polycation. Biomaterials. 1996;**17**(10):1031-1040. DOI: 10.1016/0142-9612(96)84680-1

[25] Goosen MF, O'shea GM, Sun AM, inventors; Sanofi Pasteur Ltd, assignee. Microencapsulation of living tissue and cells. United States patent US 4,806,355. 1989

[26] Blackband S, Constantinidis I, Grant S, Simpson N. NMR properties of alginate microbeads. Biomaterials. 2003;**24**:4941-4948. DOI: 10.1016/S0142-9612(03)00418-6

[27] Martinsen A et al. Alginate as immobilization material: I. Correlation between chemical and physical properties of alginate gel beads. Biotechnology and Bioengineering. 2004;**33**:79-89

[28] Saraswathi SJ, Babu B, Rengasamy R. Seasonal studies on the alginate and its biochemical composition I: *Sargassum polycystum* (Fucales), Phaeophyceae. Phycological Research. 2003;**51**(4):240-243. DOI: 10.1111/j.1440-1835.2003.t01-1-.x

[29] Sheath RG. Red Algae. Freshwater Algae of North America. 2003;**1**:197-224. DOI: 10.1016/B978-012741550-5/50006-4

[30] Qin Y. Alginate fibres: An overview of the production processes and applications in wound management. Polymer International. 2007;**57**(2):171-180. DOI: 10.1002/pi.2296

[31] Espevik T, Ostgaard K, Otterlei M, Skjak-Braek G, Soon-Shlong P, Smidsrod O. Induction of cytokine production from human monocytes stimulated with alginate. Journal of Immunotherapy. 1991;**10**:286-291. DOI: 10.1097/00002371-199108000-00007

[32] Donati I et al. New Hypothesis on the Role of Alternating Sequences in Calcium-Alginate Gels. Biomacromolecules. 2005;**6**:1031-1040. DOI: 10.1021/bm049306e

[33] Kalyani S et al. Pervaporation separation of ethanol–water mixtures through sodium alginate membranes. Desalination. 2008;**229**:68-81

[34] Holme H et al. Thermal depolymerization of alginate in the solid state. Carbohydrate Polymers. 2003. Available from: www.sciencedirect.com/science/article/pii/S0144861703001346

[35] NovaMatrix Alginate. Accessed from: http://www.novamatrix.biz/ultrapure-alginate/ [13 February 2019]

[36] Lee KY, Mooney DJ. Alginate: Properties and biomedical applications. Progress in Polymer Science. 2012;**37**(1):106-126. DOI: 10.1016/j.progpolymsci.2011.06.003

[37] Zhao X, Li J, Feng Y, Yu G, Zhou Q, He F, et al. Self-aggregation behavior of hydrophobic sodium alginate derivatives in aqueous solution and their application in the nanoencapsulation of acetamiprid. International Journal of Biological Macromolecules. 2018;**106**:418-424. DOI: 10.1016/j.ijbiomac.2017.08.038

[38] Yan J, Chen F, Amsden BG. Cell sheets prepared via gel–sol transition of calcium RGD–alginate. Acta Biomaterialia. 2016;**30**:277-284. DOI: 10.1016/j.actbio.2015.10.046

[39] Nussinovitch A. Hydrocolloid Applications: Gum Technology in the Food and Other Industries. London: Blackie Academic & Professional; 1997. DOI: 10.1007/978-1-4615-6385-3

[40] FDA Title 21-Food and Drug: Sec. 184.1724 Sodium alginate. Vol. 3. 21CFR184.1724. Available from: https://www.accessdata.fda.gov/scripts/cdrh/Cfdocs/cfCFR/CFRSearch.cfm?fr=184.1724

[41] Bixler HJ, Porse H. A decade of change in the seaweed hydrocolloids industry. Journal of Applied Phycology. 2011;**23**(3):321-335. DOI: 10.1007/s10811-010-9529-3

[42] Gibbs BF, Kermasha S, Alli I, Catherine N, Mulligan B. Encapsulation in the food industry: A review. International Journal of Food Sciences and Nutrition. 1999;**50**(3):213-224. DOI: 10.1080/096374899101256

[43] De Leo R, Quartieri A, Haghighi H, Gigliano S, Bedin E, Pulvirenti A. Application of pectin-alginate and pectin-alginate-laurolyl arginate ethyl coatings to eliminate *Salmonella enteritidis* cross contamination in egg shells. Journal of Food Safety. 2018;**38**(6):e12567. DOI: 10.1111/jfs.12567

[44] Vijayalakshmi S, Sivakamasundari SK, Moses JA, Anandharamakrishnan C. Potential application of alginates in the beverage industry. Alginates: Applications in the Biomedical and Food Industries. 2019;**13**:233-261. DOI: 10.1002/9781119487999.ch12

[45] Qin Y, Jiang J, Zhao L, Zhang J, Wang F. Applications of alginate as a functional food ingredient. In: Grumezescu A, Holban AM, eds. Biopolymers for Food Design. Cambridge: Academic Press; 2018. pp. 409-429

[46] Chang TM. Semipermeable microcapsules. Science. 1964; **146**(3643):524-525. DOI: 10.1126/science.146.3643.524

[47] Pipeleers D, Keymeulen B. Boost for alginate encapsulation in beta cell transplantation. Trends in Endocrinology & Metabolism. 2016;**27**(5):247-248. DOI: 10.1016/j.tem.2016.03.010

[48] Gonzalez-Pujana A, Orive G, Pedraz JL, Santos-Vizcaino E, Hernandez RM. Alginate microcapsules for drug delivery. In: Rehm B, Moradali M, eds. Alginates and Their Biomedical Applications. Switzerland: Springer Link; 2018. pp. 67-100. DOI: 10.1007/978-981-10-6910-9_3

[49] Omori T, Nishida T, Komoda H, Fumimoto Y, Ito T, Sawa Y, et al. A study of the xenoantigenicity of neonatal porcine islet-like cell clusters (NPCC) and the efficiency of adenovirus-mediated DAF (CD55) expression. Xenotransplantation. 2006;**13**(5):455-464. DOI: 10.1111/j.1399-3089.2006.00335.x

[50] Sandrin M, Mckenzie IF. Galα (1, 3) Gal, the major xenoantigen (s) recognized in pigs by human natural antibodies. Immunological Reviews. 1994;**141**(1):169-190. DOI: 10.1111/j.1600-065X.1994.tb00877.x

[51] McKenzie IF, Stocker J, Ting A, Morris PJ. Human lymphocytotoxic and haemagglutinating activity against sheep and pig cells. The Lancet. 1968;**292**(7564):386-387. DOI: 10.1016/S0140-6736(68)90598-9

[52] Krishnan R, Ko D, Foster CE, Liu W, Smink AM, de Haan B, et al. Immunological challenges facing translation of alginate encapsulated porcine islet xenotransplantation to human clinical trials. In: Opara E, editor. Cell Microencapsulation. Methods in Molecular Biology. New York: Humana Press; 2017. p. 305-333. DOI: 10.1007/978-1-4939-6364-5_24

[53] Safley SA, Kenyon NS, Berman DM, Barber GF, Willman M, Duncanson S, et al. Microencapsulated adult porcine islets transplanted intraperitoneally in streptozotocin-diabetic non-human primates. Xenotransplantation. 2018;**25**(6):e12450. DOI: 10.1111/xen.12450

[54] Ballios BG, Cooke MJ, van der Kooy D, Shoichet MS. A hydrogel-based stem cell delivery system to treat retinal degenerative diseases. Biomaterials. 2010;**31**(9):2555-2564. DOI: 10.1016/j.biomaterials.2009.12.004

[55] Kobayashi T, Ochi M, Yanada S, Ishikawa M, Adachi N, Deie M, et al. A novel cell delivery system using magnetically labeled mesenchymal stem cells and an external magnetic device for clinical cartilage repair. Arthroscopy: The Journal of Arthroscopic & Related Surgery. 2008;**24**(1):69-76. DOI: 10.1016/j.arthro.2007.08.017

[56] Halme DG, Kessler DA. FDA regulation of stem-cell-based therapies. The New England Journal of Medicine. 2006;**355**:1730-1735. DOI: 10.1056/NEJMhpr063086

[57] Bensaıd W, Triffitt JT, Blanchat C, Oudina K, Sedel L, Petite H. A biodegradable fibrin scaffold for mesenchymal stem cell transplantation. Biomaterials. 2003;**24**(14):2497-4502. DOI: 10.1016/S0142-9612(02)00618-X

[58] Orive G, Tam SK, Pedraz JL, Hallé JP. Biocompatibility of alginate–poly-L-lysine microcapsules for cell therapy.

Biomaterials. 2006;**27**(20):3691-3700. DOI: 10.1016/j.biomaterials.2006.02.048

[59] Orive G, Ponce S, Hernandez RM, Gascon AR, Igartua M, Pedraz JL. Biocompatibility of microcapsules for cell immobilization elaborated with different type of alginates. Biomaterials. 2002;**23**(18):3825-3831. DOI: 10.1016/S0142-9612(02)00118-7

[60] De Mesmaeker I, Robert T, Suenens KG, Stangé GM, Van Hulle F, Ling Z, et al. Increase functional β-cell mass in subcutaneous alginate capsules with porcine prenatal islet cells but loss with human adult islet cells. Diabetes. 2018;**67**(12):2640-2649. DOI: 10.2337/db18-0709

[61] Vegas AJ, Veiseh O, Gürtler M, Millman JR, Pagliuca FW, Bader AR, et al. Long-term glycemic control using polymer-encapsulated human stem cell-derived beta cells in immune-competent mice. Nature Medicine. 2016;**22**(3):306. DOI: 10.1038/nm.4030

[62] Alagpulinsa DA, Cao JJ, Driscoll RK, Sîrbulescu RF, Penson MF, Sremac M, et al. Alginate-microencapsulation of human stem cell-derived β cells with CXCL 12 prolongs their survival and function in immunocompetent mice without systemic immunosuppression. American Journal of Transplantation. 2019;**81**:32-38. DOI: 10.1111/ajt.15308

[63] Chen H, Jin S, Huang S, Folmer J, Liu J, Ge R, et al. Transplantation of alginate-encapsulated seminiferous tubules and interstitial tissue into adult rats: Leydig stem cell differentiation in vivo? Molecular and Cellular Endocrinology. 2016;**436**:250-258. DOI: 10.1016/j.mce.2016.08.046

[64] Balyura M, Gelfgat E, Ehrhart-Bornstein M, Ludwig B, Gendler Z, Barkai U, et al. Transplantation of bovine adrenocortical cells encapsulated in alginate. Proceedings of the National Academy of Sciences. 2015;**112**(8):2527-2532. DOI: 10.1073/pnas.1500242112

[65] Cacciotti I, Ceci C, Bianco A, Pistritto G. Neuro-differentiated Ntera2 cancer stem cells encapsulated in alginate beads: First evidence of biological functionality. Materials Science and Engineering: C. 2017;**81**:32-38. DOI: 10.1016/j.msec.2017.07.033

[66] Karlsson JO, Toner M. Long-term storage of tissues by cryopreservation: Critical issues. Biomaterials. 1996;**17**(3):243-256. DOI: 10.1016/0142-9612(96)85562-1

[67] Gurruchaga H, del Burgo LS, Hernandez RM, Orive G, Selden C, Fuller B, et al. Advances in the slow freezing cryopreservation of microencapsulated cells. Journal of Controlled Release. 2018;**281**:119-138. DOI: 10.1016/j.jconrel.2018.05.016

[68] Weng L, Tessier SN, Swei A, Stott SL, Toner M. Controlled ice nucleation using freeze-dried *Pseudomonas syringae* encapsulated in alginate beads. Cryobiology. 2017;**75**:1-6. DOI: 10.1016/j.cryobiol.2017.03.006

[69] Block W. Water status and thermal analysis of alginate beads used in cryopreservation of plant germplasm. Cryobiology. 2003;**47**(1):59-72. DOI: 10.1016/S0011-2240(03)00069-5

[70] Bouafia S, Jelti N, Lairy G, Blanc A, Bonnel E, Dereuddre J. Cryopreservation of potato shoot tips by encapsulation dehydration. Potato Research. 1996;**39**(1):69-78. DOI: 10.1007/BF02358208

[71] Niino T, Sakai A. Cryopreservation of alginate-coated in vitro-grown shoot tips of apple, pear and mulberry. Plant Science. 1992;**87**(2):199-206. DOI: 10.1016/0168-9452(92)90151-B

[72] Dereuddre JS, Blandin S, Hassen N. Resistance of alginate-coated somatic

embryos of carrot (*Daucus carota* L.) to desiccation and freezing in liquid nitrogen: 1. Effects of preculture. Cryo Letters. 1991;**12**:125-134

[73] Halim M, Mustafa NA, Othman M, Wasoh H, Kapri MR, Ariff AB. Effect of encapsulant and cryoprotectant on the viability of probiotic *Pediococcus acidilactici* ATCC 8042 during freeze-drying and exposure to high acidity, bile salts and heat. LWT-Food Science and Technology. 2017;**81**:210-216. DOI: 10.1016/j.lwt.2017.04.009

[74] Kanmani P, Kumar RS, Yuvaraj N, Paari KA, Pattukumar V, Arul V. Effect of cryopreservation and microencapsulation of lactic acid bacterium *Enterococcus faecium* MC13 for long-term storage. Biochemical Engineering Journal. 2011;**58**:140-147. DOI: 10.1016/j.bej.2011.09.006

[75] Capela P, Hay TK, Shah NP. Effect of cryoprotectants, prebiotics and microencapsulation on survival of probiotic organisms in yoghurt and freeze-dried yoghurt. Food Research International. 2006;**39**(2):203-211

[76] Liu X, Zhao G, Chen Z, Panhwar F, He X. Dual suppression effect of magnetic induction heating and microencapsulation on ice crystallization enables low-cryoprotectant vitrification of stem cell-alginate hydrogel constructs. ACS Applied Materials & Interfaces. 2018;**10**(19):16822-16835. DOI: 10.1021/acsbiomaterials.9b00249

[77] Zhang W, He X. Microencapsulating and banking living cells for cell-based medicine. Journal of Healthcare Engineering. 2011;**2**(4):427-446. DOI: 10.1260/2040-2295.2.4.427

[78] Kojayan GG, Alexander M, Imagawa DK, Lakey JR. Systematic review of islet cryopreservation. Islets. 2018;**10**(1):40-49. DOI: 10.1080/19382014.2017.1405202

[79] Chen W, Shu Z, Gao D, Shen AQ. Sensing and sensibility: Single-islet-based quality control assay of cryopreserved pancreatic islets with functionalized hydrogel microcapsules. Advanced Healthcare Materials. 2016;**5**(2):223-231. DOI: 10.1002/adhm.201500515

[80] Kinasiewicz J, Antosiak-Iwanska M, Godlewska E, Sitarek E, Sabat M, Fiedor P, et al. Effect of over 10-year cryopreserved encapsulated pancreatic islets of langerhans. Experimental and Clinical Transplantation: Official Journal of the Middle East Society for Organ Transplantation. 2018;**16**(4):461-465. DOI: 10.6002/ect.2016.0343

[81] Benson EE, Harding K, Ryan M, Petrenko A, Petrenko Y, Fuller B. Alginate encapsulation to enhance biopreservation scope and success: A multidisciplinary review of current ideas and applications in cryopreservation and non-freezing storage. Cryoletters. 2018;**39**(1): 14-38. Available from: https://www.ingentaconnect.com/content/cryo/cryo/2018/00000039/00000001/art00003 [Accessed: 21 March 2019]

[82] Pirnia A, Parivar K, Hemadi M, Yaghmaei P, Gholami M. Stemness of spermatogonial stem cells encapsulated in alginate hydrogel during cryopreservation. Andrologia. 2017;**49**(5):e12650. DOI: 10.1111/and.12650

[83] Swioklo S, Constantinescu A, Connon CJ. Alginate-encapsulation for the improved hypothermic preservation of human adipose-derived stem cells. Stem Cells Translational Medicine. 2016;**5**(3):339-349. DOI: 10.5966/sctm.2015-0131

[84] Gillespie LN, Zanin MP, Shepherd RK. Cell-based neurotrophin treatment supports long-term auditory neuron survival in the deaf Guinea pig. Journal of Controlled Release. 2015;**198**:26-34. DOI: 10.1016/j.jconrel.2014.11.026

[85] Dubrot J, Portero A, Orive G, Hernández RM, Palazón A, Rouzaut A, et al. Delivery of immunostimulatory monoclonal antibodies by encapsulated hybridoma cells. Cancer Immunology, Immunotherapy. 2010;**59**(11):1621-1631. DOI: 10.1007/s00262-010-0888-z

[86] Grandoso L, Ponce S, Manuel I, Arrúe A, Ruiz-Ortega JA, Ulibarri I, et al. Long-term survival of encapsulated GDNF secreting cells implanted within the striatum of parkinsonized rats. International Journal of Pharmaceutics. 2007;**343**(1-2):69-78. DOI: 10.1016/j.ijpharm.2007.05.027

[87] Joshy KS, Susan MA, Snigdha S, Nandakumar K, Laly AP, Sabu T. Encapsulation of zidovudine in PF-68 coated alginate conjugate nanoparticles for anti-HIV drug delivery. International Journal of Biological Macromolecules. 2018;**107**:929-937. DOI: 10.1016/j.ijbiomac.2017.09.078

[88] Fan L, Ge H, Zou S, Xiao Y, Wen H, Li Y, et al. Sodium alginate conjugated graphene oxide as a new carrier for drug delivery system. International Journal of Biological Macromolecules. 2016;**93**:582-590. DOI: 10.1016/j.ijbiomac.2016.09.026

[89] Yin N, Han Y, Xu H, Gao Y, Yi T, Yao J, et al. VEGF-conjugated alginate hydrogel prompt angiogenesis and improve pancreatic islet engraftment and function in type 1 diabetes. Materials Science and Engineering: C. 2016;**59**:958-964. DOI: 10.1016/j.msec.2015.11.009

[90] Ingavle GC, Gionet-Gonzales M, Vorwald CE, Bohannon LK, Clark K, Galuppo LD, et al. Injectable mineralized microsphere-loaded composite hydrogels for bone repair in a sheep bone defect model. Biomaterials. 2019;**197**:119-128. DOI: 10.1016/j.biomaterials.2019.01.005

[91] Skjåk-Bræk G, Murano E, Paoletti S. Alginate as immobilization material. II: Determination of polyphenol contaminants by fluorescence spectroscopy, and evaluation of methods for their removal. Biotechnology and Bioengineering. 1989;**33**(1):90-94

[92] Paredes Juárez GA, Spasojevic M, Faas MM, de Vos P. Immunological and technical considerations in application of alginate-based microencapsulation systems. Frontiers in Bioengineering and Biotechnology. 2014;**2**:26. DOI: 10.3389/fbioe.2014.00026

[93] Dusseault J, Tam SK, Ménard M, Polizu S, Jourdan G, Yahia LH, et al. Evaluation of alginate purification methods: Effect on polyphenol, endotoxin, and protein contamination. Journal of Biomedical Materials Research Part A. 2006;**76**(2):243-251. DOI: 10.1002/jbm.a.30541

[94] Sondermeijer HP, Witkowski P, Woodland D, Seki T, Aangenendt FJ, van der Laarse A, et al. Optimization of alginate purification using polyvinylidene difluoride membrane filtration: Effects on immunogenicity and biocompatibility of three-dimensional alginate scaffolds. Journal of Biomaterials Applications. 2016;**31**(4):510-520. DOI: 10.1177/0885328216645952

[95] Zimmermann U, ThÜrmer F, Jork A, Weber M, Mimietz S, HillgÄrtner M, et al. A novel class of amitogenic alginate microcapsules for long-term immunoisolated transplantation. Annals of the New York Academy of Sciences. 2001;**944**(1):199-215. DOI: 10.1111/j.1749-6632.2001.tb03833.x

[96] De Vos P, De Haan BJ, Wolters GH, Strubbe JH, Van Schilfgaarde R. Improved biocompatibility but limited graft survival after purification of alginate for microencapsulation of pancreatic islets. Diabetologia.

1997;**40**(3):262-270. DOI: 10.1007/s001250050673

[97] Ménard M, Dusseault J, Langlois G, Baille WE, Tam SK, Yahia LH, et al. Role of protein contaminants in the immunogenicity of alginates. Journal of Biomedical Materials Research Part B: Applied Biomaterials. 2010;**93**(2):333-340. DOI: 10.1002/jbm.b.31570

[98] De Vos P, Faas MM, Strand B. Alginate-based microcapsules for immunoisolation of pancreatic islets. Biomaterials. 2006;**27**:5603-5617. DOI: 10.1016/j.biomaterials.2006.07.010

[99] Papp G, Boros P, Nakken B, Szodoray P, Zeher M. Regulatory immune cells and functions in autoimmunity and transplantation immunology. Autoimmunity Reviews. 2017;**16**(5):435-444. DOI: 10.1016/j.autrev.2017.03.011

[100] Franz S, Rammelt S, Scharnweber D, Simon JC. Immune responses to implants—A review of the implications for the design of immunomodulatory biomaterials. Biomaterials. 2011;**32**:6692-6709. DOI: 10.1016/j.biomaterials.2011.05.078

[101] Mohammadi MR, Rodrigez S, Cao R, Alexander M, Lakey JR. Immune response to subcutaneous implants of alginate microcapsules. Materials Today: Proceedings. 2018;**5**(7):15580-15585. DOI: 10.1016/j.matpr.2018.04.166

[102] Anderson JM, Rodriguez A, Chang DT. Foreign body reaction to biomaterials. Seminars in Immunology. 2008;**20**(2):86-100. DOI: 10.1016/j.smim.2007.11.004

[103] Wynn TA, Ramalingam TR. Mechanisms of fibrosis: Therapeutic translation for fibrotic disease. Nature Medicine. 2012;**18**(7):1028. DOI: 10.1038/nm.2807

[104] De Vos P, van Hoogmoed CG, de Haan BJ, Busscher HJ. Tissue responses against immunoisolating alginate-PLL capsules in the immediate posttransplant period. Journal of Biomedical Materials Research. 2002;**62**(3):430-437. DOI: 10.1002/jbm.10345

[105] Yang D, Jones KS. Effect of alginate on innate immune activation of macrophages. Journal of Biomedical Materials Research Part A. 2009;**90**(2):411-418. DOI: 10.1002/jbm.a.32096

[106] Iwamoto Y, Xu X, Tamura T, Oda T, Muramatsu T. Enzymatically depolymerized alginate oligomers that cause cytotoxic cytokine production in human mononuclear cells. Bioscience, Biotechnology, and Biochemistry. 2003;**67**(2):258-263. DOI: 10.1271/bbb.67.258

[107] Kulseng B, Skjåk-Braek G, Følling I, Espevik T. TNF production from peripheral blood mononuclear cells in diabetic patients after stimulation with alginate and lipopolysaccharide. Scandinavian Journal of Immunology. 1996;**43**(3):335-340. DOI: 10.1046/j.1365-3083.1996.d01-43.x

[108] Jones JA, McNally AK, Chang DT, Qin LA, Meyerson H, Colton E, et al. Matrix metalloproteinases and their inhibitors in the foreign body reaction on biomaterials. Journal of Biomedical Materials Research Part A. 2008;**84**(1):158-166. DOI: 10.1002/jbm.a.31220

[109] Duvivier-Kali VF, Omer A, Parent RJ, O'Neil JJ, Weir GC. Complete protection of islets against allorejection and autoimmunity by a simple barium-alginate membrane. Diabetes. 2001;**50**(8):1698-1705. DOI: 10.2337/diabetes.50.8.1698

[110] Vishwakarma A, Bhise NS, Evangelista MB, Rouwkema J, Dokmeci MR, Ghaemmaghami AM, et al. Engineering immunomodulatory

biomaterials to tune the inflammatory response. Trends in Biotechnology. 2016;**34**(6):470-482. DOI: 10.1016/j.tibtech.2016.03.009

[111] Ricci M, Blasi P, Giovagnoli S, Rossi C, Macchiarulo G, Luca G, et al. Ketoprofen controlled release from composite microcapsules for cell encapsulation: Effect on post-transplant acute inflammation. Journal of Controlled Release. 2005;**107**(3):395-407. DOI: 10.1016/j.jconrel.2005.06.023

[112] Vernon RB, Gooden MD, Preisinger A, Gebe JA. Controlled release of monoclonal antibodies from poly-L-lysine-coated alginate spheres within a scaffolded implant mitigates autoimmune responses to transplanted islets and limits systemic antibody toxicity. Materials Science and Engineering: C. 2018;**93**:390-398. DOI: 10.1016/j.msec.2018.07.056

[113] Park HS, Kim JW, Lee SH, Yang HK, Ham DS, Sun CL, et al. Antifibrotic effect of rapamycin containing polyethylene glycol-coated alginate microcapsule in islet xenotransplantation. Journal of Tissue Engineering and Regenerative Medicine. 2017;**11**(4):1274-1284. DOI: 10.1002/term.2029

[114] Caplan AI, Correa D. The MSC: An injury drugstore. Cell Stem Cell. 2011;**9**(1):11-15. DOI: 10.1016/j.stem.2011.06.008

[115] Desai T, Shea LD. Advances in islet encapsulation technologies. Nature Reviews Drug Discovery. 2017;**16**(5):338. DOI: 10.1038/nrd.2016.232.\

[116] Follin B, Juhl M, Cohen S, Pedersen AE, Gad M, Kastrup J, et al. Human adipose-derived stromal cells in a clinically applicable injectable alginate hydrogel: Phenotypic and immunomodulatory evaluation. Cytotherapy. 2015;**17**(8):1104-1118. DOI: 10.1016/j.jcyt.2015.04.008

[117] Stucky EC, Schloss RS, Yarmush ML, Shreiber DI. Alginate micro-encapsulation of mesenchymal stromal cells enhances modulation of the neuro-inflammatory response. Cytotherapy. 2015;**17**(10):1353-1364. DOI: 10.1016/j.jcyt.2015.05.002

[118] Bloom ET. Xenotransplantation: Regulatory challenges. Current Opinion in Biotechnology. 2001;**12**(3):312-316. DOI: 10.1016/S0958-1669(00)00218-4

[119] Check E. Diabetes trial stirs debate on safety of xenotransplants. Nature. 2002;**419**:5. DOI: 10.1038/419005b

[120] US Food and Drug Administration. Guidance for Industry: Source Animal, Product, Preclinical, and Clinical Issues Concerning the Use of Xenotransplantation Products in Humans. 2003. Accessed from: http://academy.gmp-compliance.org/guidemgr/files/UCM533036.PDF [Updated: December 2016]

[121] Zhu HT, Lu L, Liu XY, Yu L, Lyu Y, Wang B. Treatment of diabetes with encapsulated pig islets: An update on current developments. Journal of Zhejiang University-Science B. 2015;**16**(5):329-343. DOI: 10.1631/jzus.B1400310

[122] Wang W, Zhaohui M, Bin Y, et al. Intra-hepatic artery transplantation of newborn porcine islets (NPI) into 20 type 1 diabetic patients with steroids immunosuppression protocol (Abstract OP-056). In: Presented at the 10th Congress of the International Pancreas and Islet Transplantation Association in Geneva 4-7 May 2005

[123] Shimoda M, Matsumoto S. Microencapsulation in clinical islet xenotransplantation. In: Cell Microencapsulation. New York, NY: Humana Press; 2017. pp. 335-345. DOI: 10.1007/978-1-4939-6364-5_25

[124] Valdes-Gonzalez R, Rodriguez-Ventura AL, White DJ,

Bracho-Blanchet E, Castillo A, Ramírez-González B, et al. Long-term follow-up of patients with type 1 diabetes transplanted with neonatal pig islets. Clinical & Experimental Immunology. 2010;**162**(3):537-542. DOI: 10.1111/j.1365-2249.2010.04273.x

[125] Valdés-González RA, Dorantes LM, Garibay GN, Bracho-Blanchet E, Mendez AJ, Dávila-Pérez R, et al. Xenotransplantation of porcine neonatal islets of Langerhans and Sertoli cells: A 4-year study. European Journal of Endocrinology. 2005;**153**(3):419-427. DOI: 10.1530/eje.1.01982

[126] Rood PP, Cooper DK. Islet xenotransplantation: Are we really ready for clinical trials? American Journal of Transplantation. 2006;**6**(6):1269-1274. DOI: 10.1111/j.1600-6143.2006.01336.x

[127] Elliott RB. Towards xenotransplantation of pig islets in the clinic. Current Opinion in Organ Transplantation. 2011;**16**(2):195-200. DOI: 10.1097/MOT.0b013e3283449dec

[128] Cooper DK, Matsumoto S, Abalovich A, Itoh T, Mourad NI, Gianello PR, et al. Progress in clinical encapsulated islet xenotransplantation. Transplantation. 2016;**100**(11):2301. DOI: 10.1097/TP.0000000000001371

[129] Barkai U, Weir GC, Colton CK, Ludwig B, Bornstein SR, Brendel MD, et al. Enhanced oxygen supply improves islet viability in a new bioartificial pancreas. Cell Transplantation. 2013;**22**(8):1463-1476. DOI: 10.3727/096368912X657341

[130] Ludwig B, Reichel A, Steffen A, Zimerman B, Schally AV, Block NL, et al. Transplantation of human islets without immunosuppression. Proceedings of the National Academy of Sciences. 2013;**110**(47):19054-19058. DOI: 10.1073/pnas.1317561110

[131] Hu Y, Zhang Z, Li Y, Ding X, Li D, Shen C, et al. Dual-crosslinked amorphous polysaccharide hydrogels based on chitosan/Alginate for wound healing applications. Macromolecular Rapid Communications. 2018;**39**(20): 1800069. DOI: 10.1002/marc.201800069

[132] McBride CA, Patel B, Stockton KA, Kapoor V, Kimble RM. Alginate dressings for donor sites of split-thickness skin grafts. Cochrane Database of Systematic Reviews. 2018;**2018**(6):1-18. DOI: 10.1002/14651858.CD013048

[133] Mir M, Ali MN, Barakullah A, Gulzar A, Arshad M, Fatima S, et al. Synthetic polymeric biomaterials for wound healing: A review. Progress in Biomaterials. 2018;**7**(1):1-21. DOI: 10.1007/s40204-018-0083-4

[134] Winters CL, Brigido SA, Liden BA, Simmons M, Hartman JF, Wright ML. A multicenter study involving the use of a human acellular dermal regenerative tissue matrix for the treatment of diabetic lower extremity wounds. Advances in Skin & Wound Care. 2008;**21**(8):375-381. DOI: 10.1097/01.ASW.0000323532.98003.26

[135] Zelen CM, FACFAS D, Kaufman J. Use of AlloPatch® Pliable, a Human Acellular Dermal Matrix, as an Adjunctive Therapy for Chronic Non-Healing Diabetic Foot Ulcers Case Studies and Clinical Review. Accessed from: https://www.mtfbiologics.org/docs/default-source/clinical/allopatch-pliable-case-studies-final-10-28-15.pdf?sfvrsn=654fe9d2_2 [Accessed: 13 March 2019]

[136] Koehler J, Brandl FP, Goepferich AM. Hydrogel wound dressings for bioactive treatment of acute and chronic wounds. European Polymer Journal. 2018;**100**:1. DOI: 10.1016/j.eurpolymj.2017.12.046

[137] Cook W. Alginate dental impression materials: Chemistry,

structure, and properties. Journal of Biomedical Materials Research. 1986;**20**(1):1-24. DOI: 10.1002/jbm.820200103

[138] Nandini VV, Venkatesh KV, Nair KC. Alginate impressions: A practical perspective. Journal of Conservative Dentistry: JCD. 2008;**11**(1):37. DOI: 10.4103/0972-0707.43416

[139] Giordano R. Impression materials: Basic properties. General Dentistry. 2000;**48**(5):510-516. Available from: http://ls-tlss.ucl.ac.uk/course-materials/DRDPDMAT_57111.pdf [Accessed: 13 March 2019]

[140] Morrow RM, Brown CE Jr, Stansbury BE, Powell JM, Rudd KD. Compatibility of alginate impression materials and dental stones. The Journal of Prosthetic Dentistry. 1971;**25**(5):556-566. DOI: 10.1016/0022-3913(71)90214-9

[141] Larsson C, von Steyern PV. Five-year follow-up of implant-supported Y-TZP and ZTA fixed dental prostheses. A randomized, prospective clinical trial comparing two different material systems. International Journal of Prosthodontics. 2010;**23**(6):5555-5561. Available from: https://www.researchgate.net/profile/Christel_Larsson2/publication/49732404_Five-Year_Follow-up_of_Implant-Supported_Y-TZP_and_ZTA_Fixed_Dental_Prostheses_A_Randomized_Prospective_Clinical_Trial_Comparing_Two_Different_Material_Systems/links/5406e7a70cf23d9765a81f93.pdf [Accessed: 15 March 2019]

[142] Pandis N, Polychronopoulou A, Eliades T. Self-ligating vs conventional brackets in the treatment of mandibular crowding: A prospective clinical trial of treatment duration and dental effects. American Journal of Orthodontics and Dentofacial Orthopedics. 2007;**132**(2):208-215. DOI: 10.1016/j.ajodo.2006.01.030

[143] Henderson NJ, Crawford PJ, Reeves BC. A randomized trial of calcium alginate swabs to control blood loss in 3-5-year-old children. British Dental Journal. 1998;**184**(4):187. DOI: 10.1038/sj.bdj.4809576

[144] O'Brien K, Lewis D, Shaw W, Combe E. A clinical trial of aligning archwires. The European Journal of Orthodontics. 1990;**12**(4):380-384. DOI: 10.1093/ejo/12.4.380

[145] Hyde TP, Craddock HL, Gray JC, Pavitt SH, Hulme C, Godfrey M, et al. A randomized controlled trial of complete denture impression materials. Journal of Dentistry. 2014;**42**(8):895-901. DOI: 10.1016/j.jdent.2014.02.005

[146] Hulme C, Yu G, Browne C, O'Dwyer J, Craddock H, Brown S, et al. Cost-effectiveness of silicone and alginate impressions for complete dentures. Journal of Dentistry. 2014;**42**(8):902-907. DOI: 10.1016/j.jdent.2014.03.001

[147] Sculean A, Auschill TM, Donos N, Brecx M, Arweiler NB. Effect of an enamel matrix protein derivative (Emdogain®) on ex vivo dental plaque vitality. Journal of Clinical Periodontology. 2001;**28**(11):1074-1078. DOI: 10.1111/j.1600-051X.2001.281113.x

[148] Tonetti MS, Lang NP, Cortellini P, Suvan JE, Adriaens P, Dubravec D, et al. Enamel matrix proteins in the regenerative therapy of deep intrabony defects: A multicentre randomized controlled clinical trial. Journal of Clinical Periodontology. 2002;**29**(4):317-325. DOI: 10.1034/j.1600-051X.2002.290407.x

[149] Froum SJ, Weinberg MA, Rosenberg E, Tarnow D. A comparative study utilizing open flap debridement with and without enamel matrix derivative in the treatment of periodontal intrabony defects: A

12-month re-entry study. Journal of Periodontology. 2001;**72**(1):25-34. DOI: 10.1902/jop.2001.72.1.25

[150] Morais JM, Papadimitrakopoulos F, Burgess DJ. Biomaterials/tissue interactions: Possible solutions to overcome foreign body response. The AAPS Journal. 2010;**12**(2):188-196. DOI: 10.1208/s12248-010-9175-3

[151] Somo SI, Langert K, Yang CY, Vaicik MK, Ibarra V, Appel AA, et al. Synthesis and evaluation of dual crosslinked alginate microbeads. Acta Biomaterialia. 2017;**65**:53-65. DOI: 10.1016/j.actbio.2017.10.046

[152] Colton CK. Oxygen supply to encapsulated therapeutic islet cells. Advanced Drug Delivery Reviews. 2014;**67-68**:93-110. DOI: 10.1016/j.addr.2014.02.007

[153] Strand BL, Coron AE, Skjak-Braek G. Current and future perspectives on Alginate encapsulated pancreatic islet. Stem Cells Translational Medicine. 2017;**6**(4):1053-1058. DOI: 10.1002/sctm.16-0116

[154] Calafiore R, Basta G. Clinical application of microencapsulated islets: Actual prospectives on progress and challenges. Advanced Drug Delivery Reviews. 2014;**67**:84-92. DOI: 10.1016/j.addr.2013.09.020

Chapter 4

The Use of Alginate Hydrogels for the Culture of Mesenchymal Stem Cells (MSCs): In Vitro and In Vivo Paradigms

Michail E. Klontzas, Hicham Drissi and Athanasios Mantalaris

Abstract

Alginate hydrogels have been widely used in stem cell cultures due to their biocompatibility, malleable nature, high water content, enhanced mass transport properties, and their functionalization with bioactive molecules providing cues that modulate cell proliferation and differentiation. Mesenchymal stem cells (MSCs) are extensively utilized in clinical cellular therapies because of their differentiation efficiency, their immunosuppressive properties, and them not being tumorigenic when implanted in vivo. MSCs are isolated from numerous fetal and adult tissues, suitable for both autologous and allogeneic applications. Consequently, alginate hydrogels/MSCs have been applied in vivo for the treatment of a wide variety of musculoskeletal, cardiac, neural, and endocrine disorders. This chapter will review the use of alginate hydrogels (physical properties and functionalization) for MSC culture in vitro (various culture systems) and the application of alginate/MSC implants (animal models and human applications) for cellular therapy purposes in vivo.

Keywords: alginate, mesenchymal stem cells, MSCs, in vivo, in vitro, hydrogels

1. Introduction

Alginate has been extensively used for tissue engineering and regenerative medicine purposes [1]. Its ability to form hydrogels under mild gelation conditions in the presence of ions such as Ca^{2+}, Ba^{2+}, and Sr^{2+} renders it suitable for cell-based applications where exposure to harsh crosslinking buffers can lead to cell damage. When alginate is exposed to a crosslinking solution, L-guluronic residues of adjacent polysaccharide strands are connected forming a hydrogel [2, 3]. Alginate hydrogels possess the advantages of natural biomaterials such as excellent biocompatibility and abundance in nature with a low cost, properties which render it an excellent candidate for cell-based regenerative medicine applications [4]. However, the lack of alginate bioactivity requires functionalization with a wide variety of molecules promoting adhesion and modulation of stem cell fate. The purpose of this chapter is to provide an overview of the use of alginate hydrogels with mesenchymal stem cells (MSCs) which represent one of the most widely used stem cell type and the only stem cell type currently in clinical use.

2. Mesenchymal stem cells (MSCs) for tissue engineering

MSCs are multipotent stem cells with the ability to proliferate and differentiate into a variety of mature cells, mainly osteocytes, chondrocytes, and adipocytes [5].

MSCs can be isolated from a multitude of adult and fetal tissues including but not limited to the bone marrow, adipose tissue, peripheral blood, synovial tissue, placenta, Wharton's jelly, and umbilical cord blood. Importantly, it has been shown that MSCs isolated from different tissue sources possess differential proliferation and differentiation capacity toward various lineages [6] (**Figure 1**). Since their description by Friedenstein et al. [7], MSCs have been evolved as the stem cell type with the most regenerative medicine applications and the only stem cell type used in clinic to date.

MSCs represent attractive stem cell candidates for the use in tissue engineering and regenerative medicine applications for a variety of reasons. Firstly, they have the ability to proliferate and differentiate producing tissues, which are clinically relevant for regenerative medicine purposes such as musculoskeletal and neural tissues. In addition, they offer the possibility of autologous use, which can avoid adverse immune responses to allogeneic cells while also possessing an immunomodulatory capacity being able to regulate the immune environment even when implanted in an allogeneic fashion. Finally, the use of MSCs avoids the ethical shortcomings of embryonic stem cell (ESC) use and is not associated with the formation of teratomas which is a characteristic of pluripotent stem cell implantation (ESCs and induced pluripotent stem cells—iPSCs) [8–10]. Recently, protocols for the derivation of MSCs from iPSCs have also enabled the production of unlimited MSC

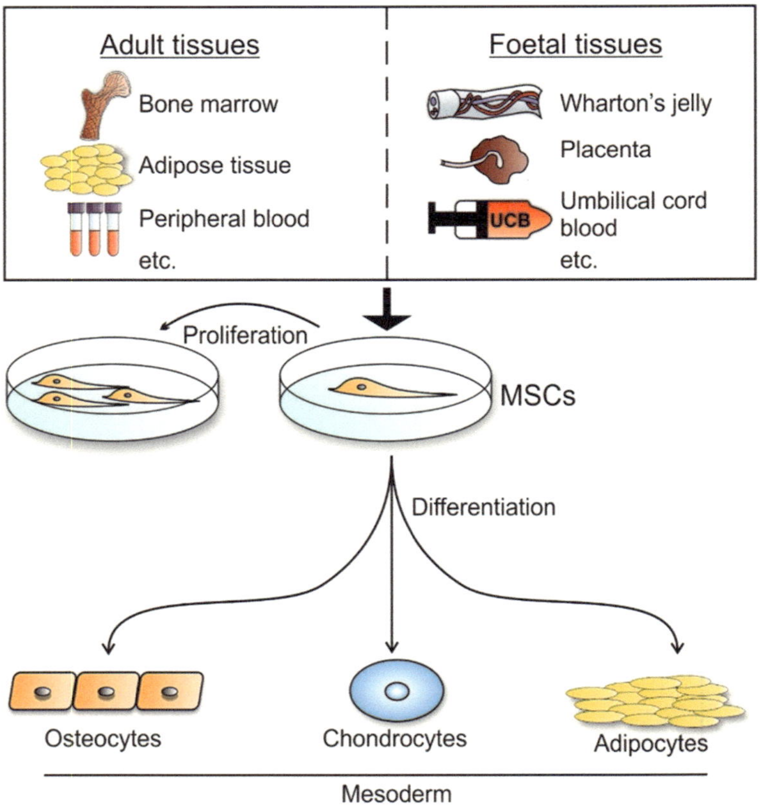

Figure 1.
Tissue sources and properties of mesenchymal stem cells.

numbers by exploiting the unlimited proliferation capacity of iPSCs prior to their differentiation to MSCs [11–13].

The use of MSCs for tissue engineering and regenerative medicine purposes requires the robust characterization of MSCs at several levels. At the moment, the International Society for Cell and Gene Therapy (ISCT) has posed the minimal criteria that need to be fulfilled so that a cell population is characterized as MSCs. These include the adherence to plastic; the presence (≥95%) of surface markers including CD73, CD90, and CD105; and the absence (≤2%) of hematopoietic markers (CD34, CD45, CD79a or CD19, CD14 or CD11b, and HLA II). Finally, cells characterized as MSCs should possess the capacity to differentiate to osteoblasts, chondroblasts, and adipocytes in vitro [14]. Other surface markers have been utilized over the years for the characterization of MSCs including Stro-1, CD271, CD146, and MSCA-1, but their use has not yet been established as a routine for MSC research [15–18]. Recently, omics strategies have emerged as promising alternatives for the comprehensive evaluation of MSC quality at the undifferentiated and differentiated states [11, 19–23].

3. The use of alginate hydrogels and MSCs in tissue engineering and regenerative medicine applications

Due to the lack of bioactive molecules on the alginate structure, alginate hydrogels used for cell-based applications require functionalization with molecules which can aid cell adhesion, increase cellular proliferation, and/or guide stem cell differentiation toward the desired cell lineages. In an attempt to increase cell adhesion on alginate hydrogels, a wide variety of extracellular matrix proteins or protein fragments have been employed. The most commonly used molecules include collagen, gelatin (product of collagen hydrolysis), and arginylglycylaspartic acid (RGD) peptide, which is the functional adhesion sequence in several extracellular matrix (ECM) proteins. Gelatin has been widely utilized for the enhancement of cell adhesion and differentiation in alginate hydrogels [24] either mixed [25] or crosslinked with alginate [26]. It has also been shown that crosslinking of alginate with gelatin reduces gelatin leak over prolonged culture while enhancing cell adhesion and vascular endothelial growth factor (VEGF) secretion compared to natural alginate and RGD-alginate [27].

Oxidized alginate has been widely used for tissue engineering purposes. Alginate can be oxidized with the use of agents including sodium permanganate ($KMnO_4$) and periodate, to produce two free aldehyde groups on the alginate backbone, offering enhanced in vitro and in vivo. Alginate oxidation is necessitated by the lack of natural alginate degrading enzymes in mammals, which is translated to a slower biodegradation of alginate hydrogels [28, 29]. Additionally, free aldehyde groups offer sites for possible crosslinking with amine group-containing molecules, which can be used for the robust functionalization of hydrogels used for tissue engineering [29, 30]. Similarly to natural alginate, a wide range of biomolecules have been used for the functionalization of oxidized alginate. The most commonly used are gelatin and RGD, which have been shown promote cell adhesion and viability [31] .

3.1 In vitro paradigms of alginate/MSC constructs

Culture of MSCs in alginate hydrogels has been attempted for applications ranging from the regeneration of bone, cartilage, and tendon to the repair of damaged myocardium and trachea. Most of the initial data on the use of alginate/MSC constructs have been obtained in vitro (**Table 1**).

Functionalization of alginate has been achieved with molecules mimicking the ECM, the most commonly used of which are RGD and gelatin. RGD has been used to increase adhesion in photo cross-linked alginate hydrogels which were found to maintain viability and promote proliferation of bone marrow MSCs [32] and muscle differentiation of umbilical cord MSCs in alginate-fibrin hydrogels [33]. Tyramine has been also cross-linked to alginate to increase MSC adhesion [34]. In hydrogels functionalized with RGD, it has been shown that high cell density favors cell-cell contact and promotes osteogenic differentiation [35] as well as increasing survival and VEGF secretion from MSC spheroids [36]. The combination of RGD with a matrix metalloproteinase cleavable peptide (proline-valine-glycine-leucine-iso-leucine-glycine) in alginate has been shown to promote adhesion and allow better

First author [reference]	Year	Type of hydrogel	MSC type
Park Y [43]	2005	Alginate	Synovial MSCs
Coates EE [42]	2013	Methacrylated alginate-HA	Bone marrow MSCs
Tohamy KM [45]	2018	Sodium alginate (SA)/hydroxyethylcellulose (HEC)/hydroxyapatite (HA)	Bone marrow MSCs
Yeatts A [60]	2011	Alginate	Bone marrow MSCs
Wang M [61]	2016	Alginate-HA	Bone marrow MSCs
Chen B [56]	2013	Strontium crosslinked alginate	Bone marrow MSCs
Weber M [41]***	2002	Alginate	C3H10T1/2 MSC cell line
Hsu S [50]	2011	Alginate/nano-sized calcium-deficient hydroxyapatite/RGD	Placental MSCs and bone marrow MSCs
Schütz K [58]	2017	Alginate/methylcellulose	Bone marrow MSCs
Kolambkar Y [64]	2007	Alginate	Amniotic fluid MSCs
Liu J [33]	2012	Alginate-fibrin-RGD	Umbilical cord MSCs
Du W-J [65]	2016	Alginate-HA	Bone marrow and adipose MSCs
Straccia M [66]	2015	Alginate-chitosan	Bone marrow MSCs
Maia F [35]	2014	Alginate-RGD	Bone marrow MSCs
Huang J [59]	2016	Alginate-gelatin-carboxymethyl chitosan	Bone marrow MSCs
Karunanithi P [38]	2016	Alginate-fucoidan	Bone marrow MSCs
Klontzas ME [20]	2019	Oxidized alginate-GHK	Umbilical cord blood MSCs
Jose S [39]	2014	Alginate-GHK	Bone marrow MSCss
Sarker B [53]	2017	Oxidized alginate-gelatin	Adipose tissue MSCs
Bernhardt A [46]	2009	Alginate-gelatin-HA	Bone marrow MSCs
Wang Y [47]	2014	Oxidized alginate-gelatin-N-succinyl chitosan	Bone marrow MSCs
Zhao L [48]	2010	Alginate-calcium phosphate	Umbilical cord MSCs
Zhou H [49]	2011	Alginate-fibrin	Umbilical cord MSCs

Table 1.
Representative in vitro studies combining alginate-based hydrogels with MSCs.

elongation of MSCs than RGD alginate [37]. Increased chondrogenesis has been also demonstrated with the incorporation of fucoidan (a heparan sulfate analogue) in alginate hydrogels seeded with bone marrow MSCs [38]. Glycine-histidine-lysine (GHK), a tripeptide fragment 0f osteonectin (a bone ECM protein), has been cross-linked with natural alginate and oxidized alginate achieving enhanced VEGF secretion from bone marrow MSCs [39] and increased osteogenic differentiation of umbilical cord blood MSCs compared to oxidized alginate with gelatin [20]. Finally, functionalization of alginate with RGD has been shown to promote adipose tissue MSC chondrogenesis via integrin-dependent transforming growth factor (TGF)-β3 activation [40].

One of the most common applications of alginate/MSC constructs is for cartilage tissue engineering. It has been shown that cells differentiated to chondroblasts in alginate hydrogels produce more collagen type II than in monolayer where they predominantly produce collagen type I [41]. In addition, photocrosslinked alginate/hyaluronic acid injectable hydrogels have been shown to support the chondrogenic differentiation of bone marrow MSCs for cartilage tissue engineering [42]. Alginate hydrogels have been also combined with synovial MSCs showing chondrogenic gene expression and collagen type II deposition under the effect of bone morphogenetic protein-2 (BMP-2). However, the authors noted that full progression of chondrogenesis was not feasible [43]. Interestingly enough when applied to bone marrow MSCs in RGD-alginate hydrogels, BMP-2 has promoted osteogenic differentiation showing that it favors osteogenic differentiation [44].

Several studies have demonstrated the suitability of alginate hydrogels in combination with MSCs for bone tissue engineering. Sodium alginate (SA)/hydroxyethylcellulose (HEC)/hydroxyapatite (HA) hydrogels have been combined with bone marrow MSCs for bone tissue engineering maintaining high cell viability and proliferation [45]. Alginate-gelatin-hydroxyapatite [46] and oxidized alginate-gelatin-N-succinyl chitosan hydrogels [47] have been shown to promote the osteogenic differentiation of bone marrow MSCs. Injectable hydrogels have been also tested for the repair of bone defects such as alginate-calcium phosphate [48] and alginate-fibrin hydrogels [49] combined with umbilical cord MSCs. Such materials enable the direct injection of the hydrogel paste in a bone defect and have been shown to promote osteogenic differentiation of MSCs facilitating fracture healing. Hydroxyapatite (calcium-deficient) and RGD have also been combined with alginate for cartilage regeneration showing that placental MSCs could perform better chondrogenesis than bone marrow MSCs [50]. However, RGD-functionalized alginate has been also shown to enhance osteogenic differentiation, mineralization, and viability [51, 52]. Oxidized alginate hydrogels have been also widely utilized for bone tissue engineering. It has been cross-linked with fibrin achieving high cell viability and osteogenic differentiation of Wharton's jelly MSCs compared to plain natural and oxidized alginate [49]. Sarker and co-workers have described the crosslinking of oxidized alginate with gelatin hydrogels for bone regeneration, demonstrating enhanced osteogenesis of adipose tissue and increase of VEGF secretion from MG-63 osteosarcoma cells compared to plain alginate and RGD-functionalized alginate [27, 53]. Other groups have also confirmed the suitability of oxidized alginate for the osteogenic differentiation of adipose-derived MSCs [53] and muscle differentiation of Wharton's jelly MSCs [54].

Apart from bone and cartilage regeneration, alginate hydrogels have found a limited number of other applications such as the regeneration of nucleus pulposus of the intervertebral disk, the cryopreservation of MSCs, and the three-dimensional printing of cellularized structures. Specifically, alginate hydrogels outperform chitosan hydrogels in glycosaminoglycan deposition and the production of collagen type II for nucleus pulposus engineering [55]. In addition, they have been used for the cryopreservation of MSCs avoiding minimizing the effects of freezing and thawing on stem cell viability [56], and various formulations of alginate such as oxidized alginate-gelatin [57], alginate/methylcellulose [58], and alginate-gelatin-carboxymethyl chitosan [59] have been found to be suitable for 3D printing applications.

Finally, it should be mentioned that there is a constantly increasing use of dynamic bioreactor cultures for the cultivation of alginate/MSC constructs. For example, dynamic perfusion bioreactor cultures of bone marrow MSCs in alginate hydrogels have been shown to enhance early in vitro osteogenic commitment and late osteogenesis [60, 61], and dynamic cultures incorporating compression forces have been used for chondrogenic differentiation purposes [62].

Despite the encouraging in vitro results, it needs to be noted that in vitro data do not necessarily correlate to the efficiency of hydrogels in vivo. As shown by Yang et al. who performed a direct in vitro-in vivo comparison of differentiation in alginate-gelatin hydrogels with MSCs, subcutaneous implantation in mice inhibits tri-lineage differentiation despite the efficient in vitro differentiation [63]. These results highlight the fact that caution is needed when extrapolating in vitro results to the in vivo setting.

3.2 In vivo paradigms of alginate/MSC constructs

Various types of alginate hydrogels have been shown to promote bone healing in animal models (**Table 2**). Injectable materials such as chitosan-alginate-BMP-2 and alginate-hydroxyapatite (HA)-mineralized microsphere combinations have been used in conjunction with MSCs to promote bone healing in vivo, demonstrating the efficient formation of trabecular bone [67, 68]. When used for bone tissue engineering, alginate hydrogels are usually seeded with MSCs and are allowed to gradually obtain higher mechanical stability as a result of ECM deposition and mineralization. However, tough alginate hydrogels have been also developed in order to achieve high mechanical stability which has been shown to promote bone healing [69]. Additionally, animal experiments have shown that when RGD is used for alginate modification, faster stress relaxation of alginate hydrogels [70] and high peptide density are linked to more efficient osteogenic differentiation than low peptide density which was linked to cell migration [71]. This correlates with results showing that increasing RGD concentrations inhibit chondrogenic differentiation in vitro [72]. Rottensteiner et al. utilized oxidized alginate-gelatin-nano-Bioglass hydrogels for bone regeneration identifying evidence of in vivo vascularization without adverse reactions, despite the cytotoxic action of Bioglass in vitro [73]. Additionally, Paul et al. successfully treated critical size calvarial defects with serum-loaded oxidized alginate-gelatin-biphasic calcium phosphate hydrogels with rat BM MSCs [74]. Importantly, encapsulation of MSCs in oxidized and natural alginate hydrogels increases vascularization which is of utmost importance in bone tissue engineering and the repair of vascular lesions [75] such as hind limb ischemia [76].

The ability of alginate hydrogels with MSCs to repair cartilage defects in animal models has been demonstrated in a variety of studies with various MSC types and hydrogel formulations. Chung et al. have compared a variety of hydrogel formulations including alginate, HA, chitosan, pluronic, and combinations of them seeded with umbilical cord blood MSCs. Their results demonstrated that even though alginate mixed with pluronic and chitosan achieved a certain degree of healing in rat knee cartilage defects, it was 4% hyaluronic acid which resulted in the optimal cartilage repair with macroscopic and microscopic appearance of adjacent healthy cartilage [77]. High-quality repair of in vivo rabbit cartilage defects has been shown with the use of

First author [reference]	Year	Type of hydrogel	MSC type	Application
Zhang F [81]	2012	Alginate	Co-culture of synovial MSCs with transgenic chondrocytes	Cartilage regeneration
Yu J [85]	2010	Alginate-RGD	Bone marrow MSCs	Myocardial regeneration
Yang C [63]	2009	Alginate-gelatin porous scaffolds	Bone marrow MSCs	Regeneration of multiple tissues
Leijs M [91]	2017	Alginate	Bone marrow MSCs	Inflammatory diseases
Steiner D [92]	2018	Oxidized alginate-gelatin	Bone marrow MSCs	Vascularization
Wang S [90]	2016	Alginate	Umbilical cord MSCs	Skin wound healing
Rottensteiner [73]	2014	Oxidized alginate with nano-Bioglass®	Bone marrow MSCs	Bone regeneration
Chung J [77]	2014	Alginate combined with pluronic, HA, and chitosan	Umbilical cord blood	Cartilage regeneration
Re'em T [84]	2012	Alginate with TGF-β1	Bone marrow MSCs	Cartilage regeneration
Sondermeijer H [86]	2018	Alginate-cyclic RGD	Bone marrow MSCs	Cardiac regeneration
Park D [67]	2005	Alginate-chitosan-BMP-2	Bone marrow MSCs	Bone regeneration
Schon LC [88]	2014	Alginate	Bone marrow MSCs	Tendon regeneration
Hashemibeni B [80]	2012	Alginate	Adipose MSCs and chondrocytes	Tracheal repair
Ho SS [93]	2016	Oxidized methacrylated alginate-RGD	Bone marrow MSCs	Bone regeneration
Moshaverinia A [89]	2014	RGD-alginate with TGF-β3	Gingival and periodontal MSCs	Tendon regeneration
Ingavle GC [68]	2019	Alginate-HA-mineralized microspheres	Bone marrow MSCs	Bone regeneration

Table 2.
Representative in vivo studies combining alginate-based hydrogels with MSCs.

bone marrow MSCs and natural alginate [78]. Alginate has been also combined with polylactic acid to promote in vivo cartilage repair with bone marrow MSCs [79]. In vivo cartilage differentiation in alginate hydrogels has been also attempted for the repair of tracheal tissue with the combination of adipose tissue MSCs and chondrocytes [80]. Synovial MSCs have also been co-cultured with chondrocytes transgenic for TGF-β3 in alginate hydrogels, demonstrating that TGF-β3 release can induce synovial MSC chondrogenesis [81]. The simultaneous activation of TGF-β3 and BMP-2 genes in MSC laden alginate hydrogels showed superior chondrogenesis compared to the isolated delivery of each one of the factors where cells progressed to endochondral osteogenesis instead of chondrogenesis [82]. Interestingly, alginate was found more capable in promoting endochondral osteogenesis than chondrogenesis when compared to chitosan [83].

Finally, TGF-β1-releasing alginate hydrogels have been used to promote chondrogenesis of MSCs, demonstrating in vitro increase of chondrogenic markers and healing of articular cartilage defects in mice [84].

Another important application of alginate/MSC constructs is the treatment of myocardial lesions. Yu et al. combined RGD-functionalized alginate hydrogels with human bone marrow MSCs showing that they could improve left ventricular function after myocardial infarction in a rat acute myocardial infarction model [85]. Cyclic RGD in alginate hydrogels has been also shown to promote neoangiogenesis and cardiac neovascularization, improving cardiac function in animals post-myocardial infarction [86]. Finally, when alginate hydrogels are used for cardiac regeneration, it has been shown that G-type alginates possess properties suited for the regeneration of cardiac tissue [87].

MSCs have been combined with alginate hydrogels for tendon repair purposes in animal model of tendon tears. For example, rat Achilles tendon lesions have been treated with hydrogels loaded with MSCs [88] showing healing of higher quality than surgical meshes and sutures. In addition, RGD-functionalized hydrogels loaded with TGF-β3 and loaded with periodontal and gingival MSCs were found to efficiently produce tendon tissue when implanted subcutaneously in mice [89].

Alginate hydrogels have also been widely utilized as wound dressings either alone or in combination with MSCs. For this application, various types of MSCs have been used including umbilical cord MSCs [90] and bone marrow MSCs in alginate-chitosan hydrogels with antibacterial properties [66].

Finally, alginate hydrogels have been used to protect MSCs from the local immune response elicited when allogeneic cells are implanted in vivo. They have been shown to provide protection from the immune system increasing the survival of MSCs in the hostile environment of the host-releasing immunomodulatory factors [91].

4. Conclusions

In conclusion, alginate/MSC constructs have been used for a wide variety of regenerative medicine applications, ranging from musculoskeletal to cardiac tissue repair. MSCs isolated from adult and fetal tissues have been combined with alginate hydrogels functionalized with extracellular matrix components, minerals, and other natural polymers and evaluated in vitro and in vivo. In vitro studies demonstrated the ability of alginate hydrogel at different formulations to support MSC growth and differentiation toward several lineages, whereas in vivo data have shown that when alginate-based materials are combined with MSCs, they can achieve successful healing of bone and cartilage defects, myocardial tissue after myocardial infarction, tendon tears, and skin wound. Nonetheless, evaluation of safety and efficacy of the constructs is required prior to clinical use. Existing in vitro and in vivo data demonstrate the potential of alginates to play an important future role in regenerative medicine, reaching the bedside and achieving regeneration of damaged tissues.

Conflict of interest

The authors declare no conflict of interest.

Author details

Michail E. Klontzas[1,2], Hicham Drissi[3] and Athanasios Mantalaris[2]*

1 Wallace H. Coulter Department of Biomedical Engineering, Biomedical Systems Engineering Laboratory, Georgia Institute of Technology, Atlanta, GA, USA

2 School of Medicine, Winship Cancer Institute, Emory University, Atlanta, GA, USA

3 Department of Orthopaedics, School of Medicine, Emory University, Atlanta, GA, USA

*Address all correspondence to: sakis.mantalaris@gatech.edu

References

[1] Lee KY, Mooney DJ. Alginate: Properties and biomedical applications. Progress in Polymer Science. 2012;**37**:106-126

[2] Sikorski P, Mo F, Skjåk-Bræk G, Stokke BT. Evidence for egg-box-compatible interactions in calcium-alginate gels from fiber X-ray diffraction. Biomacromolecules. 2007;**8**:2098-2103

[3] Kühbeck D, Mayr J, Häring M, Hofmann M, Quignard F, Díaz Díaz D. Evaluation of the nitroaldol reaction in the presence of metal ion-crosslinked alginates. New Journal of Chemistry. 2015;**39**:2306-2315

[4] Peppas NA, Hilt JZ, Khademhosseini A, Langer R. Hydrogels in biology and medicine: From molecular principles to bionanotechnology. Advanced Materials. 2006;**18**:1345-1360

[5] Pittenger MF, Mackay AM, Beck SC, Jaiswal RK, Douglas R, Mosca JD, et al. Multilineage potential of adult human mesenchymal stem cells. Science (80-). 1999;**284**:143-147

[6] Hass R, Kasper C, Böhm S, Jacobs R. Different populations and sources of human mesenchymal stem cells (MSC): A comparison of adult and neonatal tissue-derived MSC. Cell Communication and Signaling. 2011;**9**:12

[7] Friedenstein AJ, Gorskaja JF, Kulagina NN. Fibroblast precursors in normal and irradiated mouse hematopoietic organs. Experimental Hematology. 1976;**4**:267-274

[8] Seong JM, Kim B-C, Park J-H, Kwon IK, Mantalaris A, Hwang Y-S. Stem cells in bone tissue engineering. Biomedical Materials. 2010;**5**:062001

[9] Ma J, Both SK, Yang F, Cui F-Z, Pan J, Meijer GJ, et al. Concise review: Cell-based strategies in bone tissue engineering and regenerative medicine. Stem Cells Translational Medicine. 2014;**3**:98-107

[10] Klontzas ME, Kenanidis EI, Heliotis M, Tsiridis E, Mantalaris A. Bone and cartilage regeneration with the use of umbilical cord mesenchymal stem cells. Expert Opinion on Biological Therapy. 2015;**15**:1541-1552

[11] Devito L, Klontzas ME, Cvoro A, Galleu A, Simon M, Hobbs C, et al. Comparison of human isogeneic Wharton's jelly MSCs and iPSC-derived MSCs reveals differentiation-dependent metabolic responses to IFNG stimulation. Cell Death & Disease. 2019;**10**:1-13

[12] Lian Q, Zhang Y, Zhang J, Zhang HK, Wu X, Zhang Y, et al. Functional mesenchymal stem cells derived from human induced pluripotent stem cells attenuate limb ischemia in mice. Circulation. 2010;**121**:1113-1123

[13] Zhao Q, Gregory CA, Lee RH, Reger RL, Qin L, Hai B, et al. MSCs derived from iPSCs with a modified protocol are tumor-tropic but have much less potential to promote tumors than bone marrow MSCs. Proceedings of the National Academy of Sciences of the United States of America. 2015;**112**:530-535

[14] Dominici M, Le Blanc K, Mueller I, Slaper-Cortenbach I, Marini FC, Krause DS, et al. Minimal criteria for defining multipotent mesenchymal stromal cells. The International Society for Cellular Therapy Position Statement, Cytotherapy. 2006;**8**:315-317

[15] Battula VL, Treml S, Bareiss PM, Gieseke F, Roelofs H, De Zwart P, et al. Isolation of functionally distinct mesenchymal stem cell subsets using antibodies against CD56, CD271, and

mesenchymal stem cell antigen-1. Haematologica. 2009;**94**:173-184

[16] Gothard D, Greenhough J, Ralph E, Oreffo RO. Prospective isolation of human bone marrow stromal cell subsets: A comparative study between Stro-1-, CD146- and CD105-enriched populations. Journal of Tissue Engineering. 2014;**5**:1-17

[17] Bühring HJ, Battula VL, Treml S, Schewe B, Kanz L, Vogel W. Novel markers for the prospective isolation of human MSC. Annals of the New York Academy of Sciences. 2007;**1106**:262-271

[18] Bosch J, Houben AP, Radke TF, Stapelkamp D, Bünemann E, Balan P, et al. Distinct differentiation potential of "MSC" derived from cord blood and umbilical cord: Are cord-derived cells true mesenchymal stromal cells? Stem Cells and Development. 2012;**21**:1977-1988

[19] Wobma HM, Tamargo MA, Goeta S, Brown LM, Duran-Struuck R, Vunjak-Novakovic G. The influence of hypoxia and IFN-γ on the proteome and metabolome of therapeutic mesenchymal stem cells. Biomaterials. 2018;**167**:226-234

[20] Klontzas ME, Reakasame S, Silva R, Morais JCF, Vernardis S, MacFarlane RJ, et al. Oxidized alginate hydrogels with the GHK peptide enhance cord blood mesenchymal stem cell osteogenesis: A paradigm for metabolomics-based evaluation of biomaterial design. Acta Biomaterialia. 2019;**88**:224-240

[21] McNamara LE, Sjöström T, Meek RMD, Oreffo ROC, Su B, Dalby MJ, et al. Metabolomics: A valuable tool for stem cell monitoring in regenerative medicine. Journal of the Royal Society Interface. 2012;**9**:1713-1724

[22] Kalajzic I, Staal A, Yang WP, Wu Y, Johnson SE, Feyen JHM, et al. Expression profile of osteoblast lineage at defined stages of differentiation. The Journal of Biological Chemistry. 2005;**280**:24618-24626

[23] Klontzas ME, Vernardis SI, Heliotis M, Tsiridis E, Mantalaris A. Metabolomics analysis of the osteogenic differentiation of umbilical cord blood mesenchymal stem cells reveals differential sensitivity to osteogenic agents. Stem Cells and Development. 2017;**26**:723-733

[24] Venkatesan J, Bhatnagar I, Manivasagan P, Kang K-H, Kim S-K. Alginate composites for bone tissue engineering: A review. International Journal of Biological Macromolecules. 2014;**72**:269-281

[25] Hwang Y-S, Cho J, Tay F, Heng JYY, Ho R, Kazarian SG, et al. The use of murine embryonic stem cells, alginate encapsulation, and rotary microgravity bioreactor in bone tissue engineering. Biomaterials. 2009;**30**:499-507

[26] Sarker B, Papageorgiou DG, Silva R, Zehnder T, Gul-E-Noor F, Bertmer M, et al. Fabrication of alginate–gelatin crosslinked hydrogel microcapsules and evaluation of the microstructure and physico-chemical properties. Journal of Materials Chemistry B. 2014;**2**:1470

[27] Grigore A, Sarker B, Fabry B, Boccaccini AR, Detsch R. Behavior of encapsulated MG-63 cells in RGD and gelatine-modified alginate hydrogels. Tissue Engineering. Part A. 2014;**20**:2140-2150

[28] Wang L, Shansky J, Borselli C, Mooney D, Vandenburgh H. Design and fabrication of a biodegradable, covalently crosslinked shape-memory alginate scaffold for cell and growth factor delivery. Tissue Engineering. Part A. 2012;**18**:2000-2007

[29] Reakasame S, Boccaccini AR. Oxidized alginate-based hydrogels

for tissue engineering applications: A review. Biomacromolecules. 2018;**19**:3-21

[30] Balakrishnan B, Joshi N, Jayakrishnan A, Banerjee R. Self-crosslinked oxidized alginate/gelatin hydrogel as injectable, adhesive biomimetic scaffolds for cartilage regeneration. Acta Biomaterialia. 2014;**10**:3650-3663

[31] Sarker B, Singh R, Silva R, Roether JA, Kaschta J, Detsch R, et al. Evaluation of fibroblasts adhesion and proliferation on alginate-gelatin crosslinked hydrogel. PLoS One. 2014;**9**:e107952

[32] Jeon O, Alsberg E. Photo-functionalization of alginate hydrogels to promote adhesion and proliferation of human mesenchymal stem cells. Tissue Engineering. Part A. 2013;**19**:1424-1432

[33] Liu J, Zhou H, Weir MD, Xu HHK, Chen Q, Trotman CA. Fast-degradable microbeads encapsulating human umbilical cord stem cells in alginate. Tissue Engineering. Part A. 2012;**18**:2303-2314

[34] Schulz A, Gepp MM, Stracke F, Von Briesen H, Neubauer JC. Tyramine-conjugated alginate hydrogels as a platform for bioactive scaffolds. Journal of Biomedical Materials Research. Part A. 2019;**107A**:114-121

[35] Maia FR, Lourenc AH, Granja PL, Gonc RM, Barrias CC. Effect of cell density on mesenchymal stem cells aggregation in RGD-alginate 3D matrices under osteoinductive conditions. Macromolecular Bioscience. 2014;**14**:759-771

[36] Ho SS, Murphy KC, Binder BYK, Vissers CB, Leach JK. Increased survival and function of mesenchymal stem cell spheroids entrapped in instructive alginate hydrogels. Stem Cells Translational Medicine. 2016;**5**:773-781

[37] Fonseca KB, Bidarra SJ, Oliveira MJ, Granja PL, Barrias CC. Molecularly designed alginate hydrogels susceptible to local proteolysis as three-dimensional cellular microenvironments. Acta Biomaterialia. 2011;**7**:1674-1682

[38] Karunanithi P, Murali MR, Samuel S, Raghavendran HRB, Abbas AA, Kamarul T. Three dimensional alginate-fucoidan composite hydrogel augments the chondrogenic differentiation of mesenchymal stromal cells. Carbohydrate Polymers. 2016;**147**:294-303

[39] Jose S, Hughbanks ML, Binder BYK, Ingavle GC, Leach JK. Enhanced trophic factor secretion by mesenchymal stem/stromal cells with Glycine-Histidine-Lysine (GHK)-modified alginate hydrogels. Acta Biomaterialia. 2014;**10**:1955-1964

[40] Chang JC, Hsu SH, Chen DC. The promotion of chondrogenesis in adipose-derived adult stem cells by an RGD-chimeric protein in 3D alginate culture. Biomaterials. 2009;**30**:6265-6275

[41] Weber M, Steinert A, Jork A, Dimmler A, Thürmer F, Schütze N, et al. Formation of cartilage matrix proteins by BMP-transfected murine mesenchymal stem cells encapsulated in a novel class of alginates. Biomaterials. 2002;**23**:2003-2013

[42] Coates EE, Riggin CN, Fisher JP. Photocrosslinked alginate with hyaluronic acid hydrogels as vehicles for mesenchymal stem cell encapsulation and chondrogenesis. Journal of Biomedical Materials Research. Part A. 2013;**101A**:1962-1970

[43] Park Y, Sugimoto M, Watrin A, Chiquet M, Hunziker EB. BMP-2 induces the expression of chondrocyte-specific genes in bovine

synovium-derived progenitor cells cultured in three-dimensional alginate hydrogel. Osteoarthritis and Cartilage. 2005;**13**:527-536

[44] Jung T, Lee JH, Park S, Kim Y, Seo J, Shim H, et al. Effect of BMP-2 delivery mode on osteogenic differentiation of stem cells. Stem Cells International. 2017;**7859184**:1-7

[45] Tohamy KM, Mabrouk M, Soliman IE, Beherei HH, Aboelnasr MA. Novel alginate/hydroxyethyl cellulose/hydroxyapatite composite scaffold for bone regeneration: In vitro cell viability and proliferation of human mesenchymal stem cells. International Journal of Biological Macromolecules. 2018;**112**:448-460

[46] Bernhardt A, Despang F, Lode A, Demmler A, Hanke T, Gelinsky M. Proliferation and osteogenic differentiation of human bone marrow stromal cells on alginate-gelatine-hydroxyapatite scaffolds with anisotropic pore structure. Journal of Tissue Engineering and Regenerative Medicine. 2009;**3**:54-62

[47] Wang Y, Peng W, Liu X, Zhu M, Sun T, Peng Q, et al. Study of bilineage differentiation of human-bone-marrow-derived mesenchymal stem cells in oxidized sodium alginate/N-succinyl chitosan hydrogels and synergistic effects of RGD modification and low-intensity pulsed ultrasound. Acta Biomaterialia. 2014;**10**:2518-2528

[48] Zhao L, Weir MD, Xu HHK. An injectable calcium phosphate-alginate hydrogel-umbilical cord mesenchymal stem cell paste for bone tissue engineering. Biomaterials. 2010;**31**:6502-6510

[49] Zhou H, Xu HHK. The fast release of stem cells from alginate-fibrin microbeads in injectable scaffolds for bone tissue engineering. Biomaterials. 2011;**32**:7503-7513

[50] Hsu S-H, Huang T-B, Cheng S-J, Weng S-Y, Tsai C-L, Tseng C-S, et al. Chondrogenesis from human placenta-derived mesenchymal stem cells in three-dimensional. Tissue Engineering. Part A. 2011;**17**:1549-1560

[51] Evangelista MB, Hsiong SX, Fernandes R, Sampaio P, Kong HJ, Barrias CC, et al. Upregulation of bone cell differentiation through immobilization within a synthetic extracellular matrix. Biomaterials. 2007;**28**:3644-3655

[52] Bidarra SJ, Barrias CC, Barbosa MA, Soares R, Granja PL. Immobilization of human mesenchymal stem cells within RGD-grafted alginate microspheres and assessment of their angiogenic potential. Biomacromolecules. 2010;**11**:1956-1964

[53] Sarker B, Zehnder T, Rath SN, Horch RE, Kneser U, Detsch R, et al. Oxidized alginate-gelatin hydrogel: A favorable matrix for growth and osteogenic differentiation of adipose-derived stem cells in 3D. ACS Biomaterials Science & Engineering. 2017;**3**:1730-1737

[54] Baniasadi H, Mashayekhan S, Fadaoddini S, Haghirsharifzamini Y. Design, fabrication and characterization of oxidized alginate-gelatin hydrogels for muscle tissue engineering applications. Journal of Biomaterials Applications. 2016;**31**:152-161

[55] Naqvi SM, Buckley CT. Differential response of encapsulated nucleus pulposus and bone marrow stem cells in isolation and coculture in alginate and chitosan hydrogels. Tissue Engineering. Part A. 2015;**21**:288-299

[56] Chen B, Wright B, Sahoo R, Connon CJ. A novel alternative to cryopreservation for the short-term storage of stem cells for use in cell therapy using alginate encapsulation.

Tissue Engineering Part C. 2013;**19**:568-576

[57] Zehnder T, Sarker B, Boccaccini AR, Detsch R. Evaluation of an alginate-gelatine crosslinked hydrogel for bioplotting. Biofabrication. 2015;7:025001

[58] Schütz K, Placht A, Paul B, Brüggemeier S, Gelinsky M. Three-dimensional plotting of a cell-laden alginate/methylcellulose blend: Towards biofabrication of tissue engineering constructs with clinically relevant dimensions. Journal of Tissue Engineering and Regenerative Medicine. 2017;**11**:1574-1587

[59] Huang J, Fu H, Wang Z, Meng Q, Liu S, Wang H, et al. BMSCs-laden gelatin/sodium alginate/carboxymethyl chitosan hydrogel for 3D bioprinting. RSC Advances. 2016;**6**:108423-108430

[60] Yeatts AB, Fisher JP. Tubular perfusion system for the long-term dynamic culture of human mesenchymal stem cells. Tissue Engineering Part C. 2011;**17**:337-348

[61] Wang MO, Bracaglia L, Thompson JA, Fisher JP. Hydroxyapatite-doped alginate beads as scaffolds for the osteoblastic differentiation of mesenchymal stem cells. Journal of Biomedial Materials Research Part A. 2016;**104A**:2325-2333

[62] Guo T, Lim CG, Goodley AS, Xiao X, Placone JK, Ferlin KM, et al. Effect of dynamic culture and periodic compression on human Mesenchymal stem cell proliferation and chondrogenesis. Annals of Biomedical Engineering. 2016;**44**:2103-2113

[63] Yang C, Frei H, Rossi FM, Burt HM. The differential in vitro and in vivo responses of bone marrow stromal cells on novel porous gelatin–alginate scaffolds. Journal of Tissue Engineering and Regenerative Medicine. 2009;**3**:601-614

[64] Kolambkar YM, Peister A, Soker S, Atala A, Guldberg RE. Chondrogenic differentiation of amniotic fluid-derived stem cells. Journal of Molecular Histology. 2007;**38**:405-413

[65] Du W-J, Reppel L, Leger L, Schenowitz C, Huselstein C, Bensoussan D, et al. Mesenchymal stem cells derived from human bone marrow and adipose tissue maintain their immunosuppressive properties after chondrogenic differentiation. Stem Cells and Development. 2016;**25**:1454-1469

[66] Straccia MC, D'Ayala GG, Romano I, Oliva A, Laurienzo P. Alginate hydrogels coated with chitosan for wound dressing. Marine Drugs. 2015;**13**:2890-2908

[67] Park DJ, Choi BH, Zhu SJ, Huh JY, Kim BY, Lee SH. Injectable bone using chitosan-alginate gel/mesenchymal stem cells/BMP-2 composites. Journal of Cranio-Maxillofacial Surgery. 2005;**33**:50-54

[68] Ingavle GC, Gionet-Gonzales M, Vorwald CE, Bohannon LK, Clark K, Galuppo LD, et al. Injectable mineralized microsphere-loaded composite hydrogels for bone repair in a sheep bone defect model. Biomaterials. 2019;**197**:119-128

[69] Darnell MC, Sun JY, Mehta M, Johnson C, Arany PR, Suo Z, et al. Performance and biocompatibility of extremely tough alginate/polyacrylamide hydrogels. Biomaterials. 2013;**34**:8042-8048

[70] Nam S, Stowers R, Lou J, Xia Y, Chaudhuri O. Varying PEG density to control stress relaxation in alginate-PEG hydrogels for 3D cell culture studies. Biomaterials. 2019;**200**:15-24

[71] Ho SS, Keown AT, Addison B, Leach JK. Cell migration and bone formation from mesenchymal stem cell spheroids in alginate hydrogels are regulated by adhesive ligand density. Biomacromolecules. 2017;**18**:4331-4340

[72] Connelly JT, García AJ, Levenston ME. Inhibition of in vitro chondrogenesis in RGD-modified three-dimensional alginate gels. Biomaterials. 2007;**28**:1071-1083

[73] Rottensteiner U, Sarker B, Heusinger D, Dafinova D, Rath SN, Beier JP, et al. In vitro and in vivo biocompatibility of alginate dialdehyde/gelatin hydrogels with and without nanoscaled bioactive glass for bone tissue engineering applications. Materials (Basel). 2014;**7**:1957-1974

[74] Paul K, Linh NTB, Kim BR, Sarkar SK, Choi HJ, Bae SH, et al. Effect of rat bone marrow derived-stem cell delivery from serum-loaded oxidized alginate-gelatin-biphasic calcium phosphate hydrogel for bone tissue regeneration using a nude mouse critical-sized calvarial defect model. Journal of Bioactive and Compatible Polymers. 2015;**30**:188-208

[75] Steiner D, Lingens L, Fisher L, Kohn K, Detsch R, Boccaccini AR, et al. Encapsulation of mesenchymal stem cells improves vascularization of alginate-based scaffolds. Tissue Engineering. Part A. 2018;**24**:1320-1331

[76] Landázuri N, Levit RD, Joseph G, Ortega-legaspi JM, Flores CA, Weiss D, et al. Alginate microencapsulation of human mesenchymal stem cells as a strategy to enhance paracrine-mediated vascular recovery after hindlimb ischaemia. Journal of Tissue Engineering and Regenerative Medicine. 2016;**10**:222-232

[77] Chung JY, Song M, Ha C-W, Kim J-A, Lee C-H, Park Y-B. Comparison of articular cartilage repair with different hydrogel-human umbilical cord blood-derived mesenchymal stem cell composites in a rat model. Stem Cell Research & Therapy. 2014;**5**:39

[78] Dashtdar H, Rothan HA, Tay T, Ahmad RE, Ali R, Tay LX, et al. A preliminary study comparing the use of allogenic chondrogenic pre-differentiated and undifferentiated mesenchymal stem cells for the repair of full thickness articular cartilage defects in rabbits. Journal of Orthopaedic Research. 2011;**29**:1336-1342

[79] Wayne JS, McDowell CL, Shields KJ, Tuan RS. In vivo response of polylactic acid-alginate scaffolds and bone marrow-derived cells for cartilage tissue engineering. Tissue Engineering. 2005;**11**:953-963

[80] Hashemibeni B, Goharian V, Esfandiari E, Sadeghi F, Fasihi F, Alipur R, et al. An animal model study for repair of tracheal defects with autologous stem cells and differentiated chondrocytes from adipose-derived stem cells. Journal of Pediatric Surgery. 2012;**47**:1997-2003

[81] Zhang F, Su K, Fang Y, Sandhya S, Wang D-A. A mixed co-culture of mesenchymal stem cells and transgenic chondrocytes in alginate hydrogel for cartilage tissue engineering. Journal of Tissue Engineering and Regenerative Medicine. 2015;**9**:77-84

[82] Gonzalez-fernandez T, Tierney EG, Cunniffe GM, O'Brien FJ, Kelly DJ. Gene delivery of TGF-b3 and BMP2 in an MSC-laden alginate hydrogel for articular cartilage and endochondral bone tissue engineering. Tissue Engineering. Part A. 2016;**22**:776-787

[83] Sheehy EJ, Mesallati T, Vinardell T, Kelly DJ. Engineering cartilage or endochondral bone: A comparison of different naturally derived hydrogels. Acta Biomaterialia. 2015;**13**:245-253

[84] Re'em T, Kaminer-Israeli Y, Ruvinov E, Cohen S. Chondrogenesis of hMSC in affinity-bound TGF-beta scaffolds. Biomaterials. 2012;**33**:751-761

[85] Yu J, Du KT, Fang Q, Gu Y, Mihardja SS, Sievers RE, et al. The use of human mesenchymal stem cells encapsulated in RGD modified alginate microspheres in the repair of myocardial infarction in the rat. Biomaterials. 2010;**31**:7012-7020

[86] Sondermeijer HP, Witkowski P, Seki T, Van Der Laarse A, Itescu S, Hardy MA. RGDfK-peptide modified alginate scaffold for cell. Tissue Engineering. Part A. 2018;**24**:740-751

[87] Ceccaldi C, Fullana SG, Alfarano C, Lairez O, Calise D, Cussac D, et al. Alginate scaffolds for mesenchymal stem cell cardiac therapy: Influence of alginate composition. Cell Transplantation. 2012;**21**:1969-1984

[88] Schon LC, Gill N, Thorpe M, Davis J, Nadaud J, Kim J, et al. Efficacy of a mesenchymal stem cell loaded surgical mesh for tendon repair in rats. Journal of Translational Medicine. 2014;**12**:1-9

[89] Moshaverinia A, Xu X, Chen C, Ansari S, Zadeh HH, Snead ML, et al. Application of stem cells derived from the periodontal ligament or gingival tissue sources for tendon tissue regeneration. Biomaterials. 2014;**35**:2642-2650

[90] Wang S, Yang H, Tang Z, Long G, Huang W. Wound dressing model of human umbilical cord mesenchymal stem cells-alginates complex promotes skin wound healing by paracrine signaling. Stem Cells International. 2016;**3269267**:1-8

[91] Leijs MJC, Villafuertes E, Haeck JC, Koevoet WJLM, Fernandez-Gutierrez B, Hoogduijn MJ, et al. Encapsulation of allogeneic mesenchymal stem cells in alginate extends local presence and therapeutic function. European Cells & Materials. 2017;**33**:43-58

[92] Steiner D, Lingens L, Fischer L, Köhn K, Detsch R, Boccaccini AR, et al. Encapsulation of mesenchymal stem cells improves vascularization of alginate-based scaffolds. Tissue Engineering Part A. 2018;**24**:1320-1331

[93] Ho SS, Vollmer NL, Refaat MI, Jeon O, Alsberg E, et al. Bone morphogenetic protein-2 promotes human mesenchymal stem cell survival and resultant bone formation when entrapped in photocrosslinked alginate hydrogels. Advanced Healthcare Materials. 2016;**5**:2501-2509

Chapter 5

Alginate-Based Hydrogels in Regenerative Medicine

Agnieszka Kaczmarek-Pawelska

Abstract

This chapter presents the following multipotential applications of alginate-based hydrogels in tissue healing and drug delivery. It contains state of the art and summary of the literature reports, which demonstrate that alginate-based hydrogels have a great potential in tissue healing. Sodium alginate (SA) is mainly used in medical devices for healing of wounds, scars, injuries of bones, regeneration of joint cartilage, and scaffold for cell growth and in drug delivery systems (DDSs). The latest literature describes the effects of laboratory tests and in vivo, which confirm the validity of its use as a biomaterial. Alginate biodegradable scaffolds can be a template that provides a suitable substrate for cellular growth while matching the physiochemical properties of the native extracellular matrix (ECM). Matching scaffold stiffness to the surrounding tissue and optimising its rate of degradation ensure that the infiltrating cells remain viable, maintain their desired phenotype and coordinate their response over the entirety of the wound healing process.

Keywords: sodium alginate hydrogels, regenerative medicine, artificial organs, bioresorbable hydrogels, tissue healing

1. Introduction

Advances in tissue regeneration are possible due to development in the areas of engineering of the cells, materials and tissue architecture. Cell engineering mainly use genetic tools, mesenchymal stem cells or indecent pluripotent stem cells. Engineering of materials developed novel chemistries, growth factors and biomechanical conditions, whereas engineering of tissue architecture proposed novel techniques for manufacturing of scaffolds for cell growth, i.e., by using decellularised organs, 3D printing and self-assembly structures [1]. These three research areas are crucial for progress in tissue healing, and they must be compatible with each other. The stem cells will not grow properly on toxic material or in toxic biochemical and biomechanical conditions. For proper tissue healing, micromovements between the tissue structures—cells and extracellular matrix—are crucial. Like in bone growth, Wolff's law states: *If loading on a particular bone increases, the bone will remodel itself over time to become stronger to resist that sort of loading* [2, 3]. To develop new achievements in material design to improve tissue regeneration, it is necessary to analyse the interactions between the material and tissue on macro-, micro- and nanoscales. It is important to consider cell-matrix interactions and cell-cell interactions in the design and fabrication of hydrogels such as tissue engineering scaffolds because these interactions significantly affect the cell phenotype such as cell growth, adhesion and differentiation [32].

Hydrogels, as cross-linked polymeric networks, contain hydrophilic groups that promote swelling due to interaction with water. They have been in use for clinical applications since the 1960s, initially for use in ocular applications including contact lenses and intraocular lenses due to their favourable oxygen permeability and lack of irritation leading to inflammation and foreign body reaction, which was observed with other plastics. Hydrogels used in regenerative applications can be based on naturally or synthetically derived polymers. By most definitions, native tissues, particularly the extra-cellular matrix, are hydrogels and derivatives of these and other naturally based systems which are in widespread use [4, 5]. In a three-dimensional, cross-linked network of hydrophilic polymer, hydrogels offer properties such as flexibility in mechanical properties, biocompatibility, capacity to retain large ratio of solvent and ability to be prepared in an injectable form among others. These have made them as a potential candidate for use in biomedical and pharmaceutical applications such as tissue engineering [22, 24].

Molecules used for fabricating hydrogels range from natural polymers, such as dextran, gelatine and hyaluronic acid (HA), to synthetic polymers, such as polyethylene glycol (PEG), polyacrylamide (PAAm) and polyvinyl alcohol (PVA). Natural and synthetic polymers have their own advantages such as biocompatibility and high mechanical strength, respectively. Different cross-linking methods for 3D construction of hydrogel scaffolds include chemical cross-linking with covalent bond, electrostatic interaction, hydrogen bond interaction and self-assembly of polymer chains [6].

Hydrogels from natural polymers have a great potential in regenerative medicine because of their biocompatibility, biodegradability, mechanical properties, bioresorption ability and relative low cost. Among them, sodium alginate, a polysaccharide derived from brown seaweed, is widely investigated and used in biomedical applications. Alginate is highly hydrophilic and able to absorb wound exudate maintaining moist microenvironment. Alginate dressings are also useful as delivery platform in order to provide a controlled release of therapeutic substances (e.g., pain relieving and antibacterial and anti-inflammatory agents) [7], which will be discussed in the following sections.

2. Alginate hydrogels in tissue regeneration

Sodium alginate is classified in the group of hydrogels used in regenerative medicine and medical technology applications, and it is the second most abundant polysaccharide on earth, derived from seaweed, and contains β-D-mannuronate (M blocks) and β-L-guluronate subunits (G blocks) bonded with 1,4 linkage. The mechanical properties of these gels can be modulated depending on the divalent cation used to achieve cross-linking. Bivalent and trivalent cations such as Ca^{2+}, Ba^{2+}, Mg^{2+}, Fe^{2+} and Al^{3+} covalently bind alginate G blocks to form a three-dimensional structure called "egg box". For example, the use of barium or strontium instead of calcium leads to more rigid gels. M and G blocks can be combined in different sequences or alternately ensuring that bivalent cation cross-linked polymer chains form a 3D structure capable of binding large amounts of water, drugs and bioactive substances supporting tissue regeneration. Results of studies revealed that sodium alginate cross-linked with calcium ions stimulates proliferation and differentiation of osteoblasts in vitro [4, 38, 61].

2.1 Wounds and skin

As the largest organ of the human body, the skin plays a pivotal role in maintaining homeostasis as well as protecting the internal organs from the external environment. Cutaneous injuries, especially chronic wounds, burns and skin wound infections, require long-term treatment. In the United States, chronic wounds affect 6.5 million patients, with about 18% of diabetic patients over the age of 65 suffer from non-healing foot ulcers [36]. Wound healing is a complex and highly regulated physiological process that involves various cell types (i.e., immune cells, endothelial cells, keratinocytes and fibroblasts) and pathways, activated and coordinated in order to restore the tissue integrity and homeostasis [7, 8]. In the proliferation phase of a wound formation, epithelialisation occurs, and newly formed granulation tissue consisting of endothelial cells, macrophages and fibroblasts begins to cover and fill the wound area by producing new extracellular matrix (ECM). The presence of the new extracellular matrix is crucial for proper healing because it provides conditions for sustaining cells and blood vessels, which provide nutrients needed to restore the tissue integrity and homeostasis [9]. The extracellular matrix also serves as a porous and pliable scaffold for supporting the movement of cells, nutrients and growth factor through the wound environment. Studies on chemical composition of ECM during wound healing indicate that the deposition of a number of matrix components is different in chronic and acute wounds. Therefore, drug-incorporated scaffolds are particularly promising for synergistically accelerating the healing process of chronic wounds [36, 37].

Summa et al. [7] examined wound-healing potential of the hydrogel films containing sodium alginate (NaAlg) 3 g/100 ml of H_2O with the addition of 10% of the antiseptic povidone iodine (PVPI). The films were tested on a wound model on male mice, and the results showed significant reduction of the wound area and enhancement of re-epithelialisation in comparison to two groups: control and commercial products. The authors reported a significant reduction of the unhealed area after 3 days, and the wound closure was achieved within 12 days, which was more rapid and efficient than the other two groups. Histological results confirmed that NaAlg/PVPI films cause positive architectural changes on cellular level during the new tissue formation; the distance between tips of migrating epithelial tongues was the smallest in comparison to the other two groups. NaAlg/PVPI hydrogel films and their polysaccharide chains organised in a 3D structure on micro level enhance the wound healing and induce cell proliferation, whereas the presence of antiseptic povidone iodine in the films prevent bacterial infections. The authors did not examine the biomechanical properties of the NaAlg/PVPI films, so the elasticity and strength of these films are unknown, but the obtained results show that these films have biomechanical properties similar to mice skin.

Alginate-based hydrogels for wound healing with antibacterial components were also presented by Kaczmarek-Pawelska et al. [11]. Alginate hydrogel discs were obtained by cross-linking of sodium alginate solution with 0.5 M $CaCl_2$. Moreover, the researchers examined different alginate concentrations, 0.10, 0.15 and 0.20 mg/ml H_2O, and two antibacterial agents: metronidazole and silver nanoparticles (AgNP). The results showed that the obtained hydrogels have mechanical characteristics similar to the human skin, so the material is biomechanically compatible and proper for wound healing, but the value of Young modulus decreased with increasing sodium alginate concentration from 8 MPa for 0.1 mg/ml to 1.2 MPa for 0.2 mg/ml of sodium alginate. Due to the research of Edwards, the Young modulus value of the skin is from 0.3 to 30 MPa [12]. The high range of this value is caused by the individual features of the samples donor. Mechanical tests revealed that for the hydrogel samples containing silver nanoparticles, the mechanical properties are similar for each sodium alginate concentration. The difference in sodium alginate concentration determines the cross-linking level, when the cross-linking agent ($CaCl_2$) concentration is the same in every case examined. The cross-linking level influences the sample elasticity and elongation under loading. Antibacterial tests revealed that hydrogels with the addition of metronidazole and AgNP inhibits the bacterial growth after 18 h in comparison to control pure sodium alginate hydrogel. In the case of Gram-negative *Escherichia coli*, both of the aseptic additives inhibit the bacterial growth, but sodium alginate hydrogel with silver nanoparticles gives better results in tests with Gram-positive *Staphylococcus aureus*. The effectiveness of silver nanoparticles released from sodium alginate hydrogel is twice as great as metronidazole.

In the case of the sodium alginate hydrogels, the antibacterial activity and biocompatibility of the sodium alginate hydrogels also depend on the type of cation used as a cross-linking agent. Zhou et al. carried out in vitro and in vivo studies of the different cross-linking agents and examined copper, zinc, strontium and calcium ions. The results showed that zinc-cross-linked hydrogel had a spectrum of antibacterial activities, cell viability, mechanical strength and the ability of wound closure by promoting fibroblast migration, vascularisation, collagen deposition and the formation of granulation tissue. Wound healing (**Figure 1**) was compared in the six groups of rats during 21 days; it was found that ion-cross-linked hydrogels could accelerate the wound repair on rat model, especially the zinc- and strontium-cross-linked hydrogels [18].

Wichai et al. [10] proposed another wound dressing containing sodium alginate. The authors obtained membranes from bacterial cellulose (BC) incorporated with sodium alginate (AG), chitosan (CS) and copper sulphate (Cu). Moreover, they also examined how different amounts of sodium alginate and chitosan influence the membrane properties. Both of the polymers were used in different concentrations: 0.2, 0.4, 0.6, 0.8 and 1.0% w/v. The results showed that the presence of sodium alginate increased the swelling ratio, but the tensile strength decreased with high alginate concentration in the membrane. Alginate in the BC/AG composite enhanced the molecular motion of BC and perturbed the hydrogen bond of the BC composite. Furthermore, it can be as the cause of the reduced mechanical strength. Cytotoxicity of the membranes was evaluated in tests with mouse fibroblasts (L929) and human dermal fibroblasts (HDFa), in comparison to commercially available wound dressings: Acticoat®, Askina® and BluRibbon®. The results of these tests show that BC/AG/Cs-Cu composite membranes appear to display excellent antibacterial activity against *E. coli* and good biocompatibility when compared with the Acticoat®, Askina® and BluRibbon® commercial wound dressings.

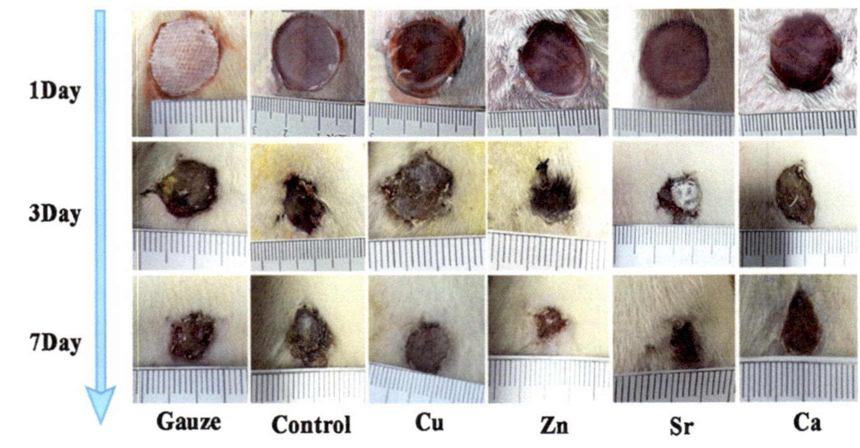

Figure 1.
The area of wound healing and general wound observation after treating with the ion-cross-linked hydrogels, nonionically cross-linked sodium alginate hydrogels such as control group and petrolatum gauze group at different times [18].

Novel dressings for skin injury healing contain alginate alone or, much more often, as a component of a multicomponent material, with, e.g., polyvinyl alcohol [13, 14, 19, 20], gelatine [13, 20], silk fibroin [15, 16], hyaluronic acid [17] or even graphene oxide [21]. These components are added to increase the mechanical properties, hydrophilicity and adhesion of the cells to the scaffolds. Moreover, to target cell response, the additives like collagen [13] and hormones such as triiodothyronine may be added [20].To support the healing process at the cellular level and recreate favourable architecture for the cell proliferation, the hydrogel scaffolds are produced by electrospinning. The high surface-to-volume ratio of nanofibers has been proven to be beneficial for the loading and delivery of drugs for wound recovery. Sobhanian [13] extracted collagen from rat tail and successfully grafted it on a nanofibrous scaffold from polyvinyl alcohol/gelatine/alginate. Modification of the scaffold with collagen increased its hydrophilicity and adhesion of the fibroblast cells. Collagen grafting resulted in the improved cell viability and proliferation on the scaffold. The obtained results confirmed that the as-prepared scaffold is hydrophilic and had acceptable bio-response and tensile properties. Tang et al. [14] produced and examined polyvinyl alcohol/alginate electrospun membrane with the addition of honey as an ancient natural wound-healing agent. The addition of honey in the nanofibers efficiently inhibited the growth of both Gram-positive bacterium (*S. aureus*) and Gram-negative bacterium (*E. coli*) and exhibited better antibacterial effect against Gram-positive bacterium than Gram-negative bacterium. Satish et al. [20] proposed a dressing for patients who suffer from chronic wounds caused by diseases such as diabetes. It is formulated in the form of a lyophilised hydrogel comprising alginate, gelatine and polyvinyl alcohol (AGP), with the aim to absorb exudates, maintain a moist environment and enhance interaction with the tissues. To enhance the healing potential of the dressing, they add triiodothyronine (active form of thyroid hormone) which plays a significant role in repair and regeneration of tissues (samples AGPT). The biomechanical properties of obtained hydrogels were proper for skin healing. Animal experiment studies (full-thickness excision wounds created in Wistar rat model) substantiated the explicit potential of the scaffold to encourage faster wound healing.

The advance in 3D bioprinting can offer precise cell patterning in predefined spatial locations, which enables the recapitulation of architectural organisation of native skin. However, the current bio-inks for skin cell printing are mostly alginate, collagen, fibrin or their mixture, which remain suboptimal [36].

2.2 Articular cartilage

Articular cartilage is a highly specialised and organised tissue that lines the ends of long bones and is integral to the functioning of all joints. It provides lubrication and mechanical strength to resist compressive and tensile forces that are essential for weight-bearing and movement. The cartilage has a unique extracellular matrix, which is comprised of an interpenetrating network of collagen and negatively charged proteoglycans and contains only one cell type—chondrocytes. Defects in cartilage do not heal properly because the cartilage has a limited regenerative capability [26]. Regeneration of articular cartilage remains an unmet medical need, which imposes a heavy burden on global economy and on the health-care community. Articular cartilage repair is still a huge challenge for researchers and clinicians. Articular cartilage defects mainly result from mechanical trauma (e.g., sports injuries). Patients with acute traumatic joint injuries have a higher chance of developing posttraumatic osteoarthritis, a degenerative condition that results in severe pain and disability, eventually requiring a total joint replacement [29]. Similar to cartilage, hydrogels retain a large portion of water, which provides lubrication and decrease of coefficient of friction (COF). The presence of water also plays an important role in the mechanical behaviour of the hydrogel structure [23].

Arjmandi and Ramezani [22] proposed and examined hybrid hydrogel-based on alginate (ALG)-polyacrylamide with the addition of silica nanoparticles (SiNP), as a candidate for cartilage replacement. They proved that its mechanical properties result from the structure of the ALG/PAAm hydrogel. The presence of covalent cross-links between two entangled polymer chains, between amine and carboxyl groups of PAAm and ALG, respectively, implies the load sharing of both networks. Alginate forms a short chain that can dissipate strain energy via recoverable breaking of ionic cross-links, meaning that after the unloading, the ionic cross-linking can be reformed, thus will be healing the damage, while the long-chained polyacrylamide network remains intact, contributing to stabilisation of the structural deformation. Moreover, the silica nanoparticles, located in a three-dimensional hydrogel structure, enhance mechanical properties and also encourage cell proliferation. Hydrogel SiNP-ALG-PAAm showed ultralow COF, coupled with high wear resistance, and tunable elastic and viscoelastic behaviour suggesting these biomaterials as promising candidates for use as a cartilage replacement.

The biomechanical properties of the hydrogels come from a combination of compositions of different factors and cross-linking levels, but they also can be determined by molecular weight and chemical properties of the hydrogel. This relationship was described by Fenbo et al. [25], Lee et al. [27] and Chen et al. [28]. It was found that hydrogels formed from alginate exhibited faster stress relaxation, which facilitated the promotion of cartilage matrix formation by chondrocytes. Moreover, 3D microenvironment, especially the elastic and relaxation moduli of the cell culture matrix, can regulate the metabolic properties of the living cells. Authors improve that molecular weight and chemical properties of the polymers used for the cell culture matrix influence on the three-dimensional cell culture system. Fenbo et al. examined high-molecular-weight alginate/chondroitin sulphate (CS) and low-molecular-weight ALG/CS (B) cross-linked by strontium. The dynamic rheology results suggest that the storage and loss moduli increase with the increase of molecular weight of alginate applied during fabrication. Cell results revealed that chondrocytes encapsulated with alginate hydrogels exhibited the best results on maintaining cell viability and inhibiting cell death [25].

Also the presence of the bioactive proteins placed in hydrogels based on sodium alginate plays a role in regeneration of the articular cartilage. Ruvinon et al. obtained injectable growth factor-loaded affinity-binding alginate hydrogel [29]. They were the first to conduct the evaluation of acellular and injectable growth factor-biomaterial combination therapy for the treatment of articular cartilage defects with a 6-month follow-up period in a large animal model. As growth factors, they use TGF-β1 and BMP-4, which were conjugated with alginate sulphate obtained from sodium alginate. Macroscopical and histological assessment of the cartilage defects treated with growth factor affinity-bound hydrogel showed effective reconstruction of articular cartilage layer, with major features of hyaline tissue, such as a glossy surface and cellular organisation. Physical nature of the applied hydrogel ensured its shear resistance, seamless integration and topographical matching to the surroundings and opposing articulating surface [29].

A great potential in articular cartilage regeneration has also a mixture of alginate with collagen as a bio-ink for 3D cell printing. Yang et al. [31] printed scaffolds and compared properties and biocompatibility in vitro of three types of the bio-ink: sodium alginate (SA) alone, sodium alginate with collagen type I (COL) and sodium alginate with agarose (AG). The results showed that the mechanical strength was improved in both SA/COL and SA/AG groups compared to SA alone. The addition of COL or AG has little impact on gelling behaviour, demonstrating the advantage as bio-inks for 3D printing. Among the three scaffolds, SA/COL could distinctly facilitate cell adhesion, accelerate cell proliferation and enhance the expression of cartilage-specific genes and may be a promising 3D bioprinting bio-ink for cartilage tissue engineering [31].

Alginate hydrogels have also a great potential in cartilage healing when mixed with hyaluronic acid [30, 32–35]. What deserves special attention is the research results. An et al. [32] presented hyaluronic acid-alginate hybrid hydrogel modified with biomimetic peptides. They enrich hydrogels with RGD peptide, which is widely used for enhancing cell-matrix interactions, and HAV peptide to increase cell-cell interactions. The authors prove that the precise control of cell-cell interactions using a scaffold is essential to regulate the cell phenotype and chondrogenic differentiation. Furthermore, the combination of these two peptides in hyaluronic acid-alginate hydrogels had a synergistic effect on the chondrogenesis of encapsulated chondrocytes, and the presented biomaterials are potentially useful for the tissue, especially cartilage regeneration [32].

2.3 Bone

The bone is a typical complex tissue with hierarchical structure that consists of approximately 70% of nano-hydroxyapatite (HA,$Ca_{10}(PO_4)6(OH_2)$) and 30% of collagen by weight. Water (with some dissolved non-collagenous organic matter) is the third elementary component. The ratio of volume and weight fractions of hydroxyapatite/collagen/water is not constant and is an individual characteristic. Among the natural polysaccharides, alginate is widely used as a biomaterial for bone tissue engineering next to chitin and chitosan. Alginate, due to it scaffold-forming ability, is a promising material for tissue engineering [38].

The biomechanical bone system is complicated; therefore, the requirements for treatment systems are high. The perfect biomaterial for bone healing should be biocompatible, have a sufficient surface area, be nontoxic with three-dimensional structure and have porosity with pore size more than 100 μm. The biomaterial should also support cell adhesion, migration and proliferation. For proper tissue growth, biomaterial should improve vascularisation that is crucial for cell migration and proliferation into the desired direction. Moreover, it should be biodegradable, be a carrier for drugs and growth factors and have mechanical properties equivalent to cortical bone [38].

Current literature report presented by Purohit et al. [39] describes fabrication of a nanocomposite scaffold of graphene oxide (GO), gelatine and alginate (GA). The properties of the obtained scaffold qualify it as a material supporting bone healing. The presence of graphene oxide in the gelatine-alginate scaffold increases its biomechanical strength. Hydrogels without the addition of graphene oxide have a compressive strength of 30 MPa, while those containing GO 44 MPa. Moreover, the presence of graphene oxides enhanced the hydrophilicity of the scaffold and provided slow degradation (~30% in 28 days). In vitro studies confirmed that an osteoblast cell line (MG-63) growth over the nanocomposite scaffolds revealed an enhancement in the cell attachment and proliferation as compared to the gelatine-alginate scaffold.

Scaffolds are crucial for bone tissue engineering since their compositions and properties could significantly affect the seeded cell behaviour. Zheng et al. [43] developed an interpenetrating network hydrogel by utilising Ca^{2+} from calcium silicate (CS) to simultaneously cross-link silk fibroin (SF) and sodium alginate. Obtained scaffolds, with different contents of calcium silicate, were systematically evaluated by physical and in vitro characterisations. Researchers found that calcium silicate inside the porous structure of hydrogel scaffolds enhance hydrophilicity, degradation, compression resistance and bioactivity. The scaffolds containing higher amount of calcium silicate have better biocompatibility and promote the osteogenic differentiation in vitro.

Sodium alginate can be easily manufactured in microspheres with three-dimensional net structures using cross-linking with calcium ions [40]. Hydrogels formed as microspheres possess some advantages for use in biomedical applications because of the larger specific surface area that can improve cell adhesion, proliferation and drug delivery. Bi et al. [40] obtained sodium alginate microspheres with the addition of chitosan (CS) and hydroxyapatite. Doxorubicin hydrochloride (Dox) was used as a drug model to study the drug loading behaviour of HA nanoparticles and hydrogel composite microspheres. In vitro examinations confirmed that the prepared HA/SA/CS/Dox drug-loaded microspheres support regeneration of the bone defects and also provide drug delivery with control of the drug release. However, the actual process of the material in vivo has not been studied. The results indicate that the hydroxyapatite/alginate hydrogel microsphere has potential in bone healing and as a drug carrier [40].

A combination of hydroxyapatite, in nano-form (nHA), and sodium alginate was also recently examined by Nabavinia et al. [45]. Nano-hydroxyapatite combined with sodium alginate showed a statistically significant impact on swelling reduction and improvement of stability and mechanical strength of hydrogels, respectively. The authors mixed SA/nHA with gelatine, to improve the cell adhesion and proliferation activities. In the research, the microcapsules were formed from solutions with a different content of each ingredient. The results show that the addition of the gelatine significantly increased swelling ratio at initial phase of incubation, similar to the degradation rate. Young modulus of the microcapsules was 0.19 MPa ± 0.02. Swelling ratio of examined hydrogel was 52% ± 8 for 24 h, and degradation rate of microspheres was 12% ± 4 (96 h). The addition of nano-hydroxyapatite in hydrogel significantly increased proliferation of the microencapsulated osteoblast cells. Examinations of cell surface receptors and protein adsorption onto hydrogel inhibit high cell proliferation and activity. The presence of gelatine in hydrogel microcapsules increases the cell proliferation, and they may be proper to build blocks for modular bone tissue [45].

Another use of the complex of sodium alginate and chitosan as a material for bone regeneration is proposed by Lee et al. [41]. The authors developed an injectable material, new calcium phosphate cement (CPC) system, incorporated with chitosan/alginate complex. Hydrogel biomaterial was produced by the interaction between cationic and anionic polymers: chitosan and alginate. In the studies, the bioactivity of cement without the polymer addition was compared with the cement containing the mixture of alginate and chitosan. Both of the cements were implanted in a rabbit femoral head defect model for 1 and 3 months. After 3 months of implantation, micro-computed tomography revealed better bone formation after implantation of cement that contains polymers than without it. The results indicate the potential value of the CPC system containing alginate-based polymer complex as an injectable bone substitute. The obtained cement system, based on chitosan/alginate mixture, may also serve as a drug carrier for faster bone healing [41].

Also a novel bone cement was presented by Shi et al. [46]. Authors use two calcium-binding agents, citric acid (CA) and sodium alginate. They were mixed with α-tricalcium phosphate (α-TCP) cement to improve the physicochemical properties of a novel biomaterial. The combination of citric acid and sodium alginate accelerated the binding of cement, increased its mechanical properties, delayed the process of hydration and prevented the formation of unclean earlandite phase. The results show that sodium alginate-citric acid hydrogel networks provided a strong cohesive action through the tight chelation with calcium ions during the hydration process of bone cements [46].

Macroporous biomaterials prepared from sodium alginate were proposed by Catanzano et al. [44] and Park et al. [42]. The first team of scientists designed natural bioactive scaffolds mimicking bone tissue. These bioactive scaffolds have to possess physicochemical properties suitable to address biological response towards newly formed bone tissues. Authors improve that the scaffold porosity and pore size play a crucial role in cell migration, adhesion and proliferation; thus they increase the cell-material surface interaction area and induce osteogenic signals transmission between cells. The authors proposed the development of macroporous alginate foams (MAFs) of porous and well-interconnected structure, useful to enhance growth and osteogenic differentiation of human mesenchymal stem cells (hMSCs) [44]. The second team [42] synthesised bio-ink, based on sodium alginate, alginate sulphate and a growth factor—bone morphogenetic protein 2. Authors used alginate sulphate, because it is a structural mimic of heparin and can strongly bind with the growth factors to prolong their activities. The exanimated mixture of alginate/alginate sulphate had good rheological properties that were not changed, after the addition of alginate sulphate, so it is proper to be used in 3D printing to obtain a structure with appropriate porosity. The bio-inks containing alginate sulphate displayed greater and more prolonged BMP-2 activities than the control bio-ink containing alginate only. Moreover, alginate/alginate sulphate bio-inks exhibited an improved retention of bone morphogenetic protein 2 in 3D-printed scaffolds. An optimal composition of alginate/alginate sulphate 3D-printed constructions to stimulate osteoblastic proliferation and differentiation in vitro is 3% alginate and 2% alginate sulphate [42].

2.4 Drug delivery

This paper describes the use of hydrogels based on sodium alginate as a material for the regeneration of specific tissues. Hydrogels were often enriched with an active substance to induce a specific tissue reaction, and they may also be classified as drug delivery systems (DDSs). But the largest group of drugs is not delivered directly to the tissue, but via oral or inhalation routes.

Poor aqueous solubility is a major problem faced in the formulation of active pharmaceutical ingredients, and it causes poor bioavailability. Although several formulation strategies have been proposed to solve this problem, a modest success has been achieved in meeting the requirements of commercially viable drug delivery systems. Therefore, extensive research on the development of optimum DDSs is still necessary. Nanoscale colloidal carrier systems developed from natural compounds such as lipids, proteins and polysaccharides for encapsulation of poorly soluble drugs have been promisingly successful recently [48].

Many drug delivery systems are still in the research phase. **Table 1** shows an overview of the latest achievements and DDSs development on the basis of sodium alginate.

A novel DDSs for pulmonary drug delivery was proposed by Athamneha et al. [47]. As the authors declare, no hybrid formulations based on hyaluronic acid and alginate have been developed for inhalation routes so far. The researchers prepared porous aerogel microspheres consisting of the mixture of alginate and hyaluronic acid. Authors examined the mixture and alginate alone to improve aerodynamic properties of microspheres, to be delivered in the lower respiratory tract. The particles were prepared via the emulsion-gelation process with subsequent supercritical CO_2 drying. Mixture of hyaluronic acid and alginate showed positive effect, prevented particle agglomeration and also improved biodegradation. The microsphere properties result from the fact that there is a hydrogen bond between carboxylate groups of ALG and the amide of the N-acetyl-D-glucosamine, which prevents the

COMPOSITION	DRUG	IN VITRO TESTS ENVIRONMENT	IN VIVO TESTS	REF.
SODIUM ALGINATE (SA)	DEXTRAMESONE	PBS	Rats	[50]
	DICLOFENAC	PBS	-	[58]
SA + MESOPOROUS SILICA	PRENDISOLONE	PBS; RWPE-1 (prostatic epithelial cells)	-	[49]
	DOXORUBICIN	PBS HELLA CELL LINE	-	[56]
SA + CHITOSAN	QUERCETIN-	PBS	-	[51]
SA + COCHLEATES	ARTEMISININ	PBS	-	[48]
SA + CHITOSAN + IRON NANOPARTICLES	DOXORUBICN	PBS HUMAN LIVING CANCER CELLS (A549)	-	[52]
SA + CHITOSAN + CELLULOSE	DEXTRAMESONE	PBS	-	[53]
SA + NANOCELLULOSE	IBUPROFEN	PBS	-	[54]
SA + LIPOSOME	DOXORUBICIN	PBS HUMAN TONQUE SQUAMOUS CELLS (CAL-27)	-	[55]
SA + GRAPHENE OXIDE + PROTEAMINE	DOXORUBICIN	MCF-7 CELLS	-	[57]
SA + OLECACID	VORICONAZOLE	HELA CELL LINE VERO CELL LINE	-	[59]
SA + POLYVINYL ALCOHOL	METFORMIN	HYDROCHLORIC ACID	-	[60]

Table 1.
Examples of tested hydrogels based on sodium alginate as drug delivery systems.

separation of components from the microsphere structure. The physicochemical and aerodynamic properties of the microspheres provided their potential suitability as a drug carrier for the pulmonary tract [47].

3. Conclusions

This chapter summarises the most frequent uses of sodium alginate in regenerative medicine and the studies on tissue regeneration. Sodium alginate is mainly used in medical devices for healing of wounds, scars, injuries of the bones, regeneration of joint cartilage, scaffolds for the cell growth and as a carrier of drug. The latest literature describes the effects of laboratory tests and in vivo, which confirm the validity of its use as a biomaterial. But there are more reports on the use of sodium alginate as a material for healing of other tissues as well. Sodium alginate is rarely used alone; most commonly it can be found in a mixture with other polymers, such as hyaluronic acid and polyvinyl alcohol, even with graphene oxide. Alginate-based hydrogels, due to their 3D polymer structure, support tissue regeneration on macro-, micro- and nanoscales. But due to its unique properties, sodium alginate is a substrate with a great potential as a hydrogel, not only in regenerative medicine but also in many different spheres of life.

Acknowledgements

This work has been financially supported by the Polish National Science Center grant 2016/21/B/ST8/01972.

Conflict of interest

The author declares that she has no conflict of interest in this publication.

Author details

Agnieszka Kaczmarek-Pawelska
Department of Biomedical Engineering, Faculty of Mechanical Engineering, University of Zielona Gora, Zielona Gora, Poland

*Address all correspondence to: a.kaczmarek@ibem.uz.zgora.pl

References

[1] Khademhosseini A, Langer R. A decade of progress in tissue engineering. Nature Protocols. 2016;**11**:1775-1781. DOI: 10.1038/nprot.2016.123

[2] Bedzinski R, Krzak-Ros J, Stefańska M, Maruszewski M. Investigation of the bone tissue and implant surface interactions. Strain. 2010;**46**:518-525. DOI: 10.1111/j.1475-1305.2007.00383.x

[3] Chen J-H, Liu C, You L, Simmons CA. Boning up on Wolff's law: Mechanical regulation of the cells that make and maintain bone. Journal of Biomechanics. 2010;**43**:108-118. DOI: 10.1016/j.jbiomech.2009.09.016

[4] Saul JM, Williams DF. Hydrogels in regenerative medicine. In: Modjarrad K, Ebnesajjad S, editors. Handbook of Polymer Applications in Medicine and Medical Devices. Elsevier; 2011. pp. 279-302. DOI: 10.1016/B978-0-323-22805-3.00012-8

[5] Palmese LL, Thapa RK, Sullivan MO, Kiick KL. Hybrid hydrogels for biomedical applications. Current Opinion in Chemical Engineering. 2019;**24**:1-15. DOI: 10.1016/j.coche.2019.02.010

[6] Wei W, Zhang Q, Zhou W, Liu Z, Wang Y, Alakpa EV, et al. Immunomodulatory application of engineered hydrogels in regenerative medicine. Applied Materials Today. 2019;**14**:126-136. DOI: 10.1016/j.apmt.2018.11.013

[7] Summa M, Russo D, Penna J, Marganoli N, Bayer JS, Bandlera T, et al. A biocompatible sodium alginate/povidone iodine film enhances wound healing. European Journal of Pharmaceutics and Biopharmaceutics. 2018;**122**:17-24. DOI: 10.1016/j.ejpb.2017.10.004

[8] Gurtner GC, Werner S, Barrandon Y, Longaker MT. Wound repair and regeneration. Nature. 2008;**453**:314-321. DOI: 10.1038/nature07039

[9] Sinno H, Prakash S. Complements and wound healing cascade: An updated review. Plastic Surgery International. 2013;**146764**:1-7. DOI: 10.1155/2013/146764

[10] Wichai S, Chuysinuan P, Chaiarwut S, Ekaburt P, Supaphol P. Development of bacterial cellulose/alginate/chitosan composites incorporating copper (II) sulfate as an antibacterial wound dressing. Journal of Drug Delivery Science and Technology. 2019;**51**:662-671. DOI: 10.1016/j.jddst.2019.03.043

[11] Kaczmarek-Pawelska A, Winiarczyk K, Mazurek J. Alginate based hydrogel for tissue regeneration: Optimization, antibacterial activity and mechanical properties. Journal of Achievements in Materials and Manufacturing Engineering. 2017;**81**:35-40. DOI: 10.5604/01.3001.0010.2034

[12] Edwards C, Marks R. Evaluation of biomechanical properties of human skin. Clinics in Dermatology. 1995;**13**:375-380. DOI: 10.1016/0738-081X(95)00078-T

[13] Sobhanian P, Khorram M, Hashemi SS, Mohammadi A. Development of nanofibrous collagen-grafted poly (vinyl alcohol)/gelatin/alginate scaffold as potential skin substitute. International Journal of Biological Macromolecules. 2019;**130**:977-987. DOI: 10.1016/j.ijbiomac.2019.03.045

[14] Tang Y, Lan X, Liang C, Zhong Z, Xie R, Zhou Y, et al. Honey loaded alginate/PVA nanofibrous membrane as a potential bioactive wound dressing. Carbohydrate Polymers. 2019;**219**:113-120. DOI: 10.1016/j.carbpol.2019.05.004

[15] Ghalei S, Nourmohammadi J, Solouk A, Mirzadem H. Enhanced cellular

response elicited by addition of amniotic fluid to alginate hydrogel-electrospun silk fibroin fibers for potential wound dressing application. Colloids and Surfaces B: Biinterfaces. 2018;**172**:82-89. DOI: 10.1016/j.colsurfb.2018.08.028

[16] Li S, Guo C, Qin H, Yu X. A promising wound dressing material with excellent cytocompatibility and proangiogenesis action for wound healing: Strontium loaded silk fibroin/sodium alginate (SF/SA) blend films. International Journal of Biological Macromolecules. 2017;**104**:969-978. DOI: 10.1016/j.ijbiomac.2017.07.020

[17] Abou-Okeil A, Fahmy HM, El-Bisi MK, Ahmed-Farid OA. Hyaluronic acid/Na-alginate films as topical bioactive wound dressings. European Polymer Journal. 2018;**109**:101-109. DOI: 10.1016/j.eurpolymj.2018.09.003

[18] Zhou Q, Kang H, Bielec M, Wu X, Cheng Q, Wei W, et al. Influence of different ions cross-linking sodium alginate-polyacrylamide hydrogels on antibacterial properties and wound healing. Carboxyhydrate Polymers. 2018;**197**:292-304. DOI: 10.1016/j.carbpol.2018.05.078

[19] Montaser AS, Rehan M, El-Naggar ME. pH-Thermosensitive hydrogel based on polyvinyl alcohol/sodium alginate/N-isopropyl acrylamide composite for treating re-infected wounds. International Journal of Biological Macromolecules. 2019;**124**:1016-1024. DOI: 10.1016/j.ijbiomac.2018.11.252

[20] Satish A, Aswathi R, Caroline Maria J, Sai Korrapati P. Triiodothyronine impregnated alginate/gelatine/polyvinyl alcohol composite scaffold designed for exudate-intensive wound therapy. European Polymer Journal. 2019;**110**:252-264. DOI: 10.1016/j.eurpolymj.2018.11.032

[21] Ma R, Wang Y, Qi H, Shi C, Wei G, Xiao L, et al. Nanocomposite sponges of sodium alginate/graphene oxide/polyvinyl alcohol as potential wound dressing: In vitro and in vivo evaluation. Composites Part B Engineering. 2019;**167**:396-405. DOI: 10.1016/j.compositesb.2019.03.006

[22] Arjmandi M, Ramezani M. Mechanical and tribological assessment of silica nanoparticle-alginatepolyacrylamide nanocomposite hydrogels as a cartilage replacement. Journal of the Mechanical Behavior of Biomedical Materials. 2019;**95**:196-204. DOI: 10.1016/j.jmbbm.2019.04.020

[23] Święszkowski W, Ku DN, Bersee HE, Kurzydłowski KJ. An elastic material for cartilage replacement in an arthritic shoulder joint. Biomaterials. 2006;**27**:1534-1541. DOI: 10.1016/j.biomaterials.2005.08.032

[24] Liu M, Zeng X, Ma C, Yi H, Ali Z, Mou X, et al. Injectable hydrogels for cartilage and bone tissue engineering. Bone Research. 2017;**5**:17014. DOI: 10.1038/boneres.2017.14

[25] Fenbo M, Xiangchao P, Bin T. Alginate/chondroitin sulfate based hybrid hydrogel with different molecular weight and its capacity to regulate chondrocytes activity. Carbohydrate Polymers. 2019;**206**:229-237. DOI: 10.1016/j.carbpol.2018.10.109

[26] Huang H, Tan Y, Ayers DC, Song J. Anionic and zwitterionic residues modulate stiffness of photo-cross-linked hydrogels and cellular behavior of encapsulated chondrocytes. ACS Biomaterials Science & Engineering. 2018;**4**:1843-1851. DOI: 10.1021/acsbiomaterials.8b00124

[27] Lee H-P, Gu L, Mooney DJ, Levenston ME, Chaudhuri O. Mechanical confinement regulates cartilage matrix formation by chondrocytes. Nature Materials. 2017;**16**:1243-1251. DOI: 10.1038/nmat4993

[28] Chen J, Irianto J, Inamdar S, Pravincumar P, Lee DA, Bader DL, et al. Cell mechanics, structure, and function are regulated by the stiffness of the three-dimensional microenvironment. Biophysical Journal. 2012;**103**:1188-1197. DOI: 10.1016/j.bpj.2012.07.054

[29] Ruvinon E, Re'em TT, Witte F, Cohen S. Articular cartilage regeneration using acellular bioactive affinity-binding alginate hydrogel: A 6-month study in a mini-pig model of osteochondral defects. Journal of Orthopaedic Translation. 2019;**16**:40-52. DOI: 10.1016/j.jot.2018.08.003

[30] Seo Y, Lee H, Lee JW, Lee KY. Hyaluronate-alginate hybrid hydrogels prepared with various linkers for chondrocyte encapsulation. Carbohydrate Polymers. 2019;**218**:1-7. DOI: 10.1016/j.carbpol.2019.04.067

[31] Yang X, Lu Z, Wu H, Li W, Zheng L, Zhao J. Collagen-alginate as bioink for three-dimensional (3D) cell printing based cartilage tissue engineering. Materials Science and Engineering: C. 2018;**83**:195-201. DOI: 10.1016/j.msec.2017.09.002

[32] An H, Lee JW, Lee HJ, Seo Y, Park H, Lee KY. Hyaluronate-alginate hybrid hydrogels modified with biomimetic peptides for controlling the chondrocyte phenotype. Carbohydrate Polymers. 2018;**197**:422-430. DOI: 10.1016/j.carbpol.2018.06.016

[33] Park H, Lee HJ, An H, Lee KY. Alginate hydrogels modified with low molecular weight hyaluronate for cartilage regeneration. Carbohydrate Polymers. 2017;**162**:100-107. DOI: 10.1016/j.carbpol.2017.01.045

[34] Chung C-W, Kang JY, Yoon I-S, Hwang H-D, Balakrishnan P, Cho H-J, et al. Interpenetrating polymer network (IPN) scaffolds of sodium hyaluronate and sodium alginate for chondrocyte culture. Colloids and Surfaces. B, Biointerfaces. 2011;**88**:711-716. DOI: 10.1016/j.colsurfb.2011.08.005

[35] Chen P, Xia C, Mo J, Mei S, Lin X, Fan S. Interpenetrating polymer network scaffold of sodium hyaluronate and sodium alginate combined with berberine for osteochondral defect regeneration. Materials Science and Engineering: C. 2018;**91**:190-200. DOI: 10.1016/j.msec.2018.05.034

[36] Kim HS, Sun X, Lee J-H, Kim H-W, Fu X, Leong KW. Advanced drug delivery systems and artificial skin grafts for skin wound healing. Advanced Drug Delivery Reviews. DOI: 10.1016/j.addr.2018.12.014

[37] Talikowska M, Fub X, Lisaka G. Application of conducting polymers to wound care and skin tissue engineering: A review. Biosensors and Bioelectronics. 2019;**135**:50-63. DOI: 10.1016/j.bios.2019.04.001

[38] Venkatesan J, Bhatnagar I, Manivasagan P, Kang K-H, Kim S-K. Alginate composites for bone tissue engineering: A review. International Journal of Biological Macromolecules. 2015;**72**:269-281. DOI: 10.1016/j.ijbiomac.2014.07.008

[39] Purohit SD, Bhaskar R, Singh H, Yadav I, Kumar Gupta M, Chandra Mishra N. Development of a nanocomposite scaffold of gelatin-alginate-graphene oxide for bone tissue engineering. International Journal of Biological Macromolecules. 2019;**133**:592-602. DOI: 10.1016/j.ijbiomac.2019.04.113

[40] Bi Y-g, Lin Z-t, Deng S-t. Fabrication and characterization of hydroxyapatite/sodium alginate/chitosan composite microspheres for drug delivery and bone tissue engineering. Materials Science and Engineering: C. 2019;**100**:576-583. DOI: 10.1016/j.msec.2019.03.040

[41] Lee H-J, Kim B, Padalhin AR, Lee B-T. Incorporation of chitosan-alginate complex into injectable calcium phosphate cement system as a bone graft material. Materials Science and Engineering: C. 2019;**94**:385-392. DOI: 10.1016/j.msec.2018.09.039

[42] Park J, Lee SJ, Lee H, Park SA, Lee JY. Three dimensional cell printing with sulfated alginate for improved bone morphogenetic protein-2 delivery and osteogenesis in bone tissue engineering. Carbohydrate Polymers. 2018;**196**:217-224. DOI: 10.1016/j.carbpol.2018.05.048

[43] Zheng A, Cao L, Liu Y, Wu J, Zeng D, Hu L, et al. Biocompatible silk/calcium silicate/sodium alginate composite scaffolds for bone tissue engineering. Carbohydrate Polymers. 2018;**199**:244-255. DOI: 10.1016/j.carbpol.2018.06.093

[44] Catanzano O, Soriente A, La Gatta A, Cammarota M, Ricci G, Fasolino I, et al. Macroporous alginate foams crosslinked with strontium for bone tissue engineering. Carbohydrate Polymers. 2018;**202**:72-83. DOI: 10.1016/j.carbpol.2018.08.086

[45] Nabavinia M, Baradar Khoshfetrat A, Naderi-Meshkin H. Nano-hydroxyapatite-alginate-gelatin microcapsule as a potential osteogenic building block for modular bone tissue engineering. Materials Science and Engineering: C. 2019;**97**:67-77. DOI: 10.1016/j.msec.2018.12.033

[46] Shi H, Zhang W, Liu X, Zeng S, Yu T, Zhou C. Synergistic effects of citric acid—sodium alginate on physicochemical properties of α-tricalcium phosphate bone cement. Ceramics International. 2019;**45**:2146-2152. DOI: 10.1016/j.ceramint.2018.10.124

[47] Athamneha T, Amina A, Benkec E, Ambrusc R, Leopold CS, Gurikova P, et al. Alginate and hybrid alginate-hyaluronic acid aerogel microspheres as potential carrier for pulmonary drug delivery. Journal of Supercritical Fluids. 2019;**150**:49-55. DOI: 10.1016/j.supflu.2019.04.013

[48] Shuddhodana JZ. Alginate-coating of artemisinin-loaded cochleates results in better control over gastro-intestinal release for effective oral delivery. Journal of Drug Delivery Science and Technology. 2019;**52**:27-36. DOI: 10.1016/j.jddst.2019.04.020

[49] de Lima HHC, Kupfer VL, Moisés MP, Guilherme MR, Rinaldi J d C, Felisbino SL, et al. Bionanocomposites based on mesoporous silica and alginate for enhanced drug delivery. Carbohydrate Polymers. 2018;**196**:126-134. DOI: 10.1016/j.carbpol.2018.04.107

[50] Zhang R, Lei L, Song Q, Li X. Calcium ion cross-linking alginate/dexamethasone sodium phosphate hybrid hydrogel for extended drug release. Colloids and Surfaces. B, Biointerfaces. 2019;**175**:569-575. DOI: 10.1016/j.colsurfb.2018.11.083

[51] Nalini T, Khaleel Basha S, Majeeth Mohamed Sadiq A, Sugantha Kumari V, Kaviyarasu K. Development and characterization of alginate/chitosan nanoparticulate system for hydrophobic drug encapsulation. Journal of Drug Delivery Science and Technology. 2019;**52**:65-72. DOI: 10.1016/j.jddst.2019.04.002

[52] Xie M, Zhang F, Peng H, Zhang Y, Li Y, Xu Y, et al. Layer-by-layer modification of magnetic graphene oxide by chitosan and sodium alginate with enhanced dispersibility for targeted drug delivery and photothermal therapy. Colloids and Surfaces. B, Biointerfaces. 2019;**76**:462-470. DOI: 10.1016/j.colsurfb.2019.01.028

[53] Jeddi MK, Mahkam M. Magnetic nano carboxymethyl cellulose alginate/chitosan hydrogel beads as

biodegradable devices for controlled drug delivery. International Journal of Biological Macromolecules. 2019;**135**:829-838. DOI: 10.1016/j.ijbiomac.2019.05.210

[54] Supramaniam J, Adnan R, Kaus NHM, Bushr R. Magnetic nanocellulose alginate hydrogel beads as potential drug delivery system. International Journal of Biological Macromolecules. 2018;**118**:640-648. DOI: 10.1016/j.ijbiomac.2018.06.043

[55] Shtenberg Y, Goldfeder M, Prinz H, Shainsky J, Ghantous Y, Abu El-Naaj I, et al. Mucoadhesive alginate pastes with embedded liposomes for local oral drug delivery. International Journal of Biological Macromolecules. 2018;**111**:62-69. DOI: 10.1016/j.ijbiomac.2017.12.137

[56] Yuan N, Li S, Li G. Sodium alginate coated mesoporous silica for dual bio-responsive controlled drug delivery. Journal of Drug Delivery Science and Technology. 2018;**46**:348-353. DOI: 10.1016/j.jddst.2018.05.026

[57] Xie M, Zhang F, Liu L, Zhang Y, Li Y, Li H, et al. Surface modification of graphene oxide nanosheets by protamine sulfate/sodium alginate for anti-cancer drug delivery application. Applied Surface Science. 2018;**440**:853-860. DOI: 10.1016/j.apsusc.2018.01.175

[58] Ghosal K, Das A, Sanjoy Das SK, Mahmood S, Ramadan MAM, Thomas S. Synthesis and characterization of interpenetrating polymeric networks based bio-composite alginate film: A well-designed drug delivery platform. International Journal of Biological Macromolecules. 2019;**130**:645-654. DOI: 10.1016/j.ijbiomac.2019.02.117

[59] Querobino SM, de Fariab NC, Vigatob AA, da Silvac BGM, Machadod IP, Costac MS, et al. Sodium alginate in oil-poloxamer organogels for intravaginal drug delivery: Influence on structural parameters, drug release mechanisms, cytotoxicity and in vitro antifungal activity. Materials Science and Engineering: C. 2019;**99**:1350-1361. DOI: 10.1016/j.msec.2019.02.036

[60] Martínez-Gómez F, Guerrero J, Matsuhiro B, Pavez J. In vitro release of metformin hydrochloride from sodium alginate/polyvinyl alcohol hydrogels. Carbohydrate Polymers. 2017;**155**:182-191. DOI: 10.1016/j.carbpol.2016.08.079

[61] Wang Y. Programmable hydrogels. Biomaterials. 2018;**178**:663-680. DOI: 10.1016/j.biomaterials.2018.03.008

Chapter 6

Role of Alginates Combined with Natural Extracts to Prevent the Gastric Acid-Related Damage

Francesca Uberti, Lorenzo Secondini, Ian Stoppa, Mietta Catera and Claudio Molinari

Abstract

The human stomach is extremely vulnerable to various attacks able to cause erosion and mucosal epithelium damage which lead to gastrointestinal tract bleeding and/or ulcer perforations and finally worsen the original disease. A prolonged exposition to strong acidic environment causes coagulation necrosis resulting from the desiccating action of the acid on proteins in exposed tissues with inflammation and accumulation of intracellular radical oxygen species. Therapeutic strategies aim to treat both symptoms and epithelial damage with chemical or mechanical approaches. In this context, alginates seem to have great importance, especially if combined with other molecules known to have some properties on gastric epithelial cells, for example, vitamin D3, extract of prickly pear and olive leaves, and a tyndalized probiotic. This natural composition is able to exert a gastroprotective effect to maintain or restore the integrity of gastric epithelium through an antioxidant pathway, inhibiting apoptosis and activating survival kinases better than other pharmacological or natural active principles.

Keywords: alginates, vitamin D3, prickly pear, olive leaves, tyndalized probiotic

1. Introduction

The impact of gastric diseases on human health is a worldwide problem in modern society [1, 2]. For example, in the USA, studies have reported gastrointestinal illness rates in the range of 0.5–2 episodes/year/person and incidence of 5–100 episodes/1000/week according to seasons and age. The number of episodes of gastrointestinal illnesses is similar in both 40-year-old studies and in recent ones [3, 4]. The gastrointestinal disorder, including chronic gastritis, duodenal and gastric ulceration, adenocarcinoma, and gastric mucosa-associated lymphoid tissue (MALT), may have a common cause which is gastroesophageal reflux disease (GERD). The cardinal symptom is heartburn caused by the involuntary movement of gastric contents to the esophagus that occurs several times a day, mainly in postprandial period [5]. In particular, most reflux episodes are of short duration, asymptomatic, and limited to the distal esophagus [6]. However, some episodes occur with typical symptoms such as burning sensation in the chest that can also extend to the throat, gastric pain, episodes of regurgitation, dysphagia, and sensation of bolus in the throat [7]. One of the risk factors is bad eating habits that can aggravate gastroesophageal reflux and can contribute to the delayed gastric emptying with an increase of acid secretion in the stomach [8]. In the human stomach, the acid environment (pH 1 to 2) acts both as a primary defense against infections and intervenes in the early stages of digestion [9]. The gastrointestinal epithelium is a fundamental barrier protecting the gastrointestinal mucosa from damage through the ability of epithelial cells to spread and migrate across the basement membrane to repair the damage [4]. However, gastric acid (HCl) secreted from gastric parietal cells has been reported to determine gastric mucosal injuries, and, consequently, a prolonged exposition to strong acidic environment causes coagulation necrosis in exposed tissues [10]. A mild gastritis condition can cause long-lasting damage resulting in cellular injury which in turn causes inflammation [11] that creates further free radical-dependent tissue destruction [12, 13]. This injury involves DNA and can lead to stomach cancer genesis [14]. Some recent studies have shown that non-steroidal anti-inflammatory drugs (NSAIDs) are one of the most common causes of damage on the gastric mucosa through the production of free oxygen radicals (ROS) leading to lipid peroxidation and apoptosis [10, 15] of cells. In particular, superoxide anion (O^{-2}) produced by mitochondria is the main cause of oxidative damage [16] and plays a critical role in the pathogenesis of gastric disorders [17]. Around 30 million people consume NSAIDs globally every day [18] since they are prescribed because of their efficacy in the management of pain, inflammation, and fever [19]. Adverse effects associated with NSAIDs, such as alterations in renal function, effects on blood pressure, hepatic injury, and platelet inhibition, are a challenge in clinical treatment optimization [20]. However, gastric mucosal perforation and bleeding are a major concern as well as the worst outcome of prolonged NSAID therapy [21]. NSAIDs are able to induce gastric mucosal lesions because of their acidic properties [22]. The mechanism behind gastric damage involves a highly acidic gastric environment that favors the migration of nonionized lipophilic NSAIDs into the epithelial cells [23]. Diclofenac is the most widely prescribed NSAID for treating pain, inflammation, and several forms of cancer [24, 25]. The main clinical problem exerted by diclofenac is toxicity related to oxidative injury of tissues, which appears to play a role in the pathophysiology of digestive tract ulceration [18, 25, 26]. For this reason, in order to prevent the damage, NSAID treatments are usually associated to proton-pump inhibitors (PPI) [27]. However, the anatomical and functional integrity of gastric mucosa rely on the balance between aggressive and defensive mechanisms [19]; for this reason, the success of pharmacological treatments in prevention or healing of gastric lesions depends both on the blockade of acid secretion and on the enhancement of mucosal protective factors [19]. In addition, current evidence suggests that PPI are also associated with numerous side effects such as hypergastrinemia, enteric infections, adverse cardiovascular events, and increased mortality rates [23]. Basing on these data, it can therefore be assumed that gastric acid can induce ROS production, lipid peroxidation, and apoptosis through a mechanism similar to that observed by NSAIDs [10]. For this reason, ROS, including H_2O_2, are a major cause of cellular oxidative damage [16], and they play a critical role in the pathogenesis of gastric disorders [2, 17]. After a gastric mucosa damage, several events occur in order to restore the integrity of the layer; normal epithelial repair consists of restitution of functions and regeneration of anatomical integrity involving epithelial proliferation followed by a remodeling phase [28]. During restitution, epithelial cells spread through the basement membrane to restore cell continuity, a process that is independent of cell proliferation. The clinical need to prevent or restore the damage of gastric mucosa in early stage encourages the search of novel agents able to counteract both the adverse effects of drugs and hyperacidic conditions with a better safety profile, in particular using natural compounds. A new group of widely used molecules includes alginates, a polymer of alginic acid derived from the cell wall of various brown algae. Alginate-based compounds have been available for several decades [29] and are listed as inactive ingredients with a substantial and independent benefit from alginate formulation [29]. Recently, there is a new growing interest in alginates as a therapy for GERD, including patients with continued symptoms despite acid suppression therapy [30]. Alginates are polysaccharides composed of two β-d-mannuronic acid (M) and α-1-glucuronic acid (G) monomers which are held together by β 1,4 bonds; these monomers are not organized in repeated units, and they can be considered as a set of heterogeneous molecules since they are distributed as several different repetitions called M, G, or MG blocks [31, 32]. These alginates are able to block the HCl reflux in a mechanic manner; indeed, they do not have any pharmacologic property [33]. The mechanism of action of alginates has been called "rafting", which means that in the presence of gastric acid, they form a gel in which carbon dioxide (resulting from the splitting of bicarbonate) is trapped. Then the gel is carried to the top of the gastric contents neutralizing the acidity and preventing the ascent of acid material into the esophagus [34]. The advantage of alginate-based reflux suppressants over antacid alone is that they provide rapid and longer-lasting symptom relief [35].

Subsequently, it was seen that it is useful to associate alginates with natural substances. This association has been found to be effective in promoting stomach health, reducing inflammation, and supporting the immune system. Zinc, a micronutrient involved in multiple functions, is able to act as a coenzyme on several enzymes that protect cells against free radical damage [36]. Furthermore, zinc has direct effects against inflammation, as it helps to stabilize the membrane of mast cells, responsible for inflammation [37]. Other natural products with antioxidant property seem to play an active role in the stomach well-being, such as blueberries or licorice, that they are able to reduce the production of cytokines and at the same time to increase the production of the mucous membrane of the stomach [38]. Moreover alginate/antacid system has been used as a carrier of probiotic, drugs, and plant extracts [39]. For example, alginate/bicarbonate combined with two herbal gastroprotective extracts (*Opuntia ficus-indica* and *Olea europaea*) has been successfully evaluated in patients with GERD [39]. However, the most common treatments for gastroesophageal reflux includes different molecules such as magnesium hydroxide or aluminum hydroxide (commercially named Maalox®) in which they absorb gastric acidity, reducing the pH and reducing/reversibly blocking acid secretion by parietal cells. The effectiveness of these preparations is due to their ability to exert a buffering effect on the gastric pH [40], but the adverse effect is that they can cause an accumulation of aluminum which is a common cause of neurodegeneration and neurotoxicity [40].

Recent studies have explored a possible role of vitamin D_3, the active form of vitamin D, on gastroprotection as one of the extra skeletal effects this vitamin has [4, 23]. Vitamin D_3 binds its receptor VDR which is present in several tissue targets in the digestive system, in particular in the oral region, and in epithelial cells of the oral cavity, tongue, and gums. In addition, vitamin D_3 appears to have a therapeutic role in gastric mucosa as well, stimulating cell proliferation and differentiation [41] and regulating endocrine/paracrine gastrin and pepsinogen secretions [42]. Finally, vitamin D_3 acts on smooth muscle cells in the pyloric region and in different areas of the small intestine [42]. Furthermore, the low plasmatic level of vitamin D_3 is found to be responsible for an insufficient emptying of the stomach, swelling, constipation, and intestinal irritation [42]. After the binding between vitamin D_3 and its receptor, several intracellular events involved in different mechanism start, including the protective role against oxidative stress [43], the regulation of autophagic pathways through the regulation of ATG16L1, a protein complex necessary for autophagy [44], and the ability to inhibit apoptosis by increasing the expression of endothelial nitric oxide synthase (eNOS) leading to the nitric oxide (NO) production [43]. In this context, vitamin D_3 can exert some beneficial effects on gastric tissue. For this reason, its use in association with other gastroprotective agents such as alginates can increase therapeutic efficacy of the formulation in respect to the efficacy that would be obtained only with gastroprotective drugs. Indeed, this effect is described in a recent study in which this association (vitamin D_3 and raft-forming alginates, buffers, polysaccharides, and biophenols named Aquilea Reflux®) could be of greater efficacy when compared to other gastroprotectants (e.g., Maalox® or Gaviscon®) or other natural extracts (e.g., Neobianacid®) [4, 23]. Aquilea Reflux® is a dietary supplement that combines the properties of calcium alginate in a buffer solution, resulting from alkaline salts useful to counteract situations of high acidity, with a tyndalized probiotic (Pylopass®) and an extract of prickly pear and olive leaves (Mucosave®). The extract of prickly pear is useful for its emollient and soothing characteristics at the level of the digestive system. All these agents were added to vitamin D_3. This study demonstrates for the first time that the combination between alginate-based gastroprotector agent and vitamin D_3 has a beneficial effect joining the effects of a mechanical barrier with the modulation of intracellular pathways in order to maintain or restore the integrity of gastric epithelium. Indeed, Aquilea Reflux® is able to improve the adhesivity of cells which is crucial on cell migration involving two important extracellular matrix glycoproteins, vitronectin and fibronectin. This is more important because it indicates that vitamin D_3 is able to improve the beneficial effects induced by alginates, thus supporting data about the mechanism of gastroprotection induced by alginates [45]. Another important element is a time of adhesion, which is an important reparative event; the combination is able to occur rapidly, confirming other data about the reparative events following acute gastric injury [46]. Since there is evidence that oxidative stress plays an important role in the pathogenesis of acute gastric injury [47–49], Aquilea Reflux® has been also tested to verify if it is able to improve both cell viability and cell proliferation after H_2O_2 or HCl exposure. This combination significantly reduced ROS production and decreased cell viability loss, suggesting that cell damage and cytotoxicity can be reduced.

These results suggest that it may exert a better gastroprotective effect through an antioxidant pathway, inhibiting apoptosis and activating survival kinases. Such effect was stronger in preventing epithelial damage than what was observed using other gastroprotective agents such as Gaviscon®, Maalox®, or proton-pump inhibitors. Ultimately, it can be said that alginate-based gastroprotectors combined with vitamin D_3 have beneficial properties on gastric epithelial cells, joining the effects of a mechanical barrier with the modulation of intracellular pathways in order to maintain or restore the integrity of gastric epithelium. In addition, comparing the activity to other natural products, such as Neobianacid® which is a mixture of polysaccharides and flavonoids able to improve the protection of the stomach and the esophagus thanks to the presence of Poliprotect® and a flavonoid fraction (*Matricaria recutita* and *Glycyrrhiza glabra*), the combination composed of alginates plus vitamin D3 appears to have significant effects. Indeed, this combination significantly reduced ROS production and decreased cell viability loss after the injury, suggesting that cell damage and cytotoxicity can be prevented, exerting a better gastroprotective effect through an antioxidant pathway, inhibiting apoptosis, and activating survival kinases. Such effect was stronger in preventing epithelial damage than what was observed using other gastroprotective agents such as Neobianacid® (**Figure 1**).

These data show that it is possible to improve the beneficial effects of alginates by combining active ingredients that are capable of intervening at the cellular

DOI: http://dx.doi.org/10.5772/intechopen.88135

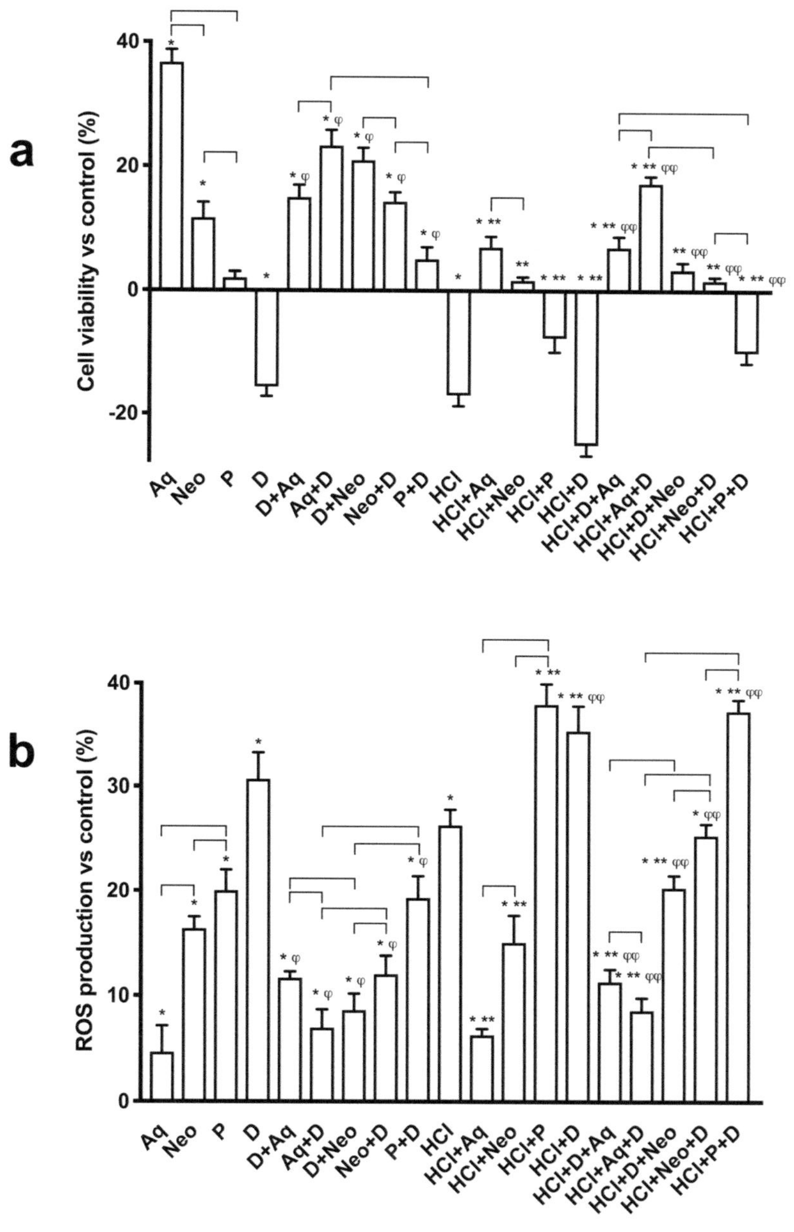

Figure 1.
*Effects of Aq and Neo alone and combined with diclofenac during acidic and hyperacidic conditions. In panel A cell viability and in panel B ROS production observed in gastric epithelial cells treated for 24 h. P= pantoprazole, D= diclofenac. The other abbreviations are similarly reported in the figure. Data are expressed as means ± SD (%) of five independent experiments normalized to control values. *p < 0.05 vs. control; **p < 0.05 vs. HCl; φp < 0.05 vs. diclofenac; φφp < 0.05 vs. HCl + diclofenac; arrows indicate p < 0.05 between different groups.*

level to improve viability and to reduce the production of ROS, from which significant damage to the gastric mucosa originates. The formulation called Aquilea Reflux®, with its combination of chemical, mechanical, and biological agents, has proven to be effective in preventing cellular alterations caused by NSAIDs in both acid and hyperacidic conditions, reducing ROS production and apoptotic mechanism, and increasing the activation of survival kinases and cell proliferation.

2. Conclusions

In conclusion it can be stated that the antacid and gastroesophageal reflux abilities of alginate-based preparations could be significantly improved by combining natural extraction components and vitamin D3, providing an association of chemical, mechanical, and cellular action to achieve a complete protective effect.

Acknowledgements

This study was partially supported by AGING Project, Dipartimento di Eccellenza.

Laborest Spa contributed by supplying the tested chemical substances.

Conflict of interest

Lorenzo Secondini and Mietta Catera are employees of Laborest Spa; however, they provide an unbiased contribution to this study.

Acronyms and abbreviations

HCl	gastric acid
GERD	gastroesophageal reflux disease
NSAID	non-steroidal anti-inflammatory drugs
PPI	proton-pump inhibitors
ROS	free oxygen radicals
eNOS	endothelial nitric oxide synthase
NO	nitric oxide

Author details

Francesca Uberti[1]*, Lorenzo Secondini[2], Ian Stoppa[1], Mietta Catera[2] and Claudio Molinari[1]

1 Physiology Laboratory, Department of Translational Medicine, UPO, Novara, Italy

2 Laborest Italia S.r.l., Gruppo Uriach, Assago Milan Italy

*Address all correspondence to: francesca.uberti@med.uniupo.it

References

[1] Boland CR, Luciani MG, Gasche C, Goel A. Infection, inflammation, and gastrointestinal cancer. Gut. 2005;**54**:1321-1331

[2] Hu XT, Ding C, Zhou N, Xu C. Quercetin protects gastric epithelial cell from oxidative damage in vitro and in vivo. European Journal of Pharmacology. 2015;**754**:115-124. DOI: 10.1016/j.ejphar.2015.02.007

[3] Payment P, Hunter PR. Endemic and epidemic infectious intestinal disease and its relationship to drinking water. In: Fewtrell L, Bartram J, editors. Water Quality: Guidelines, Standards and Health. London: IWA Publishing; 2001. pp. 61-88

[4] Uberti F, Bardelli C, Morsanuto V, Ghirlanda S, Molinari C. Role of vitamin D(3) combined to alginates in preventing acid and oxidative injury in cultured gastric epithelial cells. BMC Gastroenterology. 2016;**16**(1):127. DOI: 10.1186/s12876-016-0543-z

[5] Marseglia L, Manti S, D'Angelo G, Gitto E, Salpietro C, Centorrino A, et al. Gastroesophageal reflux and congenital gastrointestinal malformations. World Journal of Gastroenterology. 2015;**21**(28):8508-8515. DOI: 10.3748/wjg.v21.i28.8508

[6] Vandenplas Y, Hassall E. Mechanisms of gastroesophageal reflux and gastroesophageal reflux disease. Journal of Pediatric Gastroenterology and Nutrition. 2002;**35**(2):119-136

[7] Galmiche JP, Clouse RE, Bálint A, Cook IJ, Kahrilas PJ, Paterson WG, et al. Functional esophageal disorders. Gastroenterology. 2006;**130**(5):1459-1465. DOI: 10.1053/j.gastro.2005.08.060

[8] Argyrou A, Legaki E, Koutserimpas C, Gazouli M, Papaconstantinou I, Gkiokas G, et al. Risk factors for gastroesophageal reflux disease and analysis of genetic contributors. World Journal of Clinical Cases. 2018;**6**(8):176-182. DOI: 10.12998/wjcc.v6.i8.176

[9] Sun Z, Liu H, Yang Z, Shao D, Zhang W, Ren Y, et al. Intestinal trefoil factor activates the PI3K/Akt signaling pathway to protect gastric mucosal epithelium from damage. International Journal of Oncology. 2014;**45**(3):1123-1132. DOI: 10.3892/ijo.2014.2527

[10] Matsui H, Nagano Y, Shimokawa O, Kaneko T, Rai K, Udo J, et al. Gastric acid induces mitochondrial superoxide production and lipid peroxidation in gastric epithelial cells. Journal of Gastroenterology. 2011;**46**:1167-1176. DOI: 10.1007/s00535-011-0434-6

[11] Davidson G, Kritas S, Butler R. Stressed mucosa. Nestlé Nutrition Workshop Series. Paediatric Programme. 2007;**59**:133-142. DOI: 10.1159/000098532

[12] Boeckxstaens GE. Neuroimmune interaction in the gut: From bench to bedside. Verhandelingen - Koninklijke Academie voor Geneeskunde van België. 2006;**68**:329-335

[13] Iezzi A, Ferri C, Mezzetti A, Cipollone F. COX-2: Friend or foe? Current Pharmaceutical Design. 2007;**13**:1715-1721

[14] Fox JG, Wang TC. Inflammation, atrophy, and gastric cancer. The Journal of Clinical Investigation. 2007;**117**:60-69. DOI: 10.1172/JCI30111

[15] Murphy MP, Smith RA. Drug delivery to mitochondria: The key to mitochondrial medicine. Advanced Drug Delivery Reviews. 2000;**41**(2):235-250

[16] Brand MD, Buckingham JA, Esteves TC, Green K, Lambert AJ, Miwa S,

et al. Mitochondrial superoxide and aging: Uncoupling-protein activity and superoxide production. Biochemical Society Symposium. 2004;**71**:203-213

[17] Bhattacharyya A, Chattopadhyay R, Mitra S, Crowe SE. Oxidative stress: An essential factor in the pathogenesis of gastrointestinal mucosal diseases. Physiological Reviews. 2014;**94**(2):329-354. DOI: 10.1152/physrev.00040.2012

[18] Mazumder S, De R, Sarkar S, Siddiqui AA, Saha SJ, Banerjee C, et al. Selective scavenging of intra-mitochondrial superoxide corrects diclofenac-induced mitochondrial dysfunction and gastric injury: A novel gastroprotective mechanism independent of gastric acid suppression. Biochemical Pharmacology. 2016;**121**:33-51. DOI: 10.1016/j.bcp.2016.09.027

[19] Fornai M, Natale G, Colucci R, Tuccori M, Carazzina G, Antonioli L, et al. Mechanisms of protection by pantoprazole against NSAID-induced gastric mucosal damage. Naunyn-Schmiedeberg's Archives of Pharmacology. 2005;**372**(1):79-87

[20] Gadzhanova S, Ilomäki J, Roughead EE. COX-2 inhibitor and non-selective NSAID use in those at increased risk of NSAID-related adverse events: A retrospective database study. Drugs & Aging. 2013;**30**(1):23-30. DOI: 10.1007/s40266-012-0037-9

[21] Sostres C, Gargallo CJ, Lanas A. Nonsteroidal anti-inflammatory drugs and upper and lower gastrointestinal mucosal damage. Arthritis Research & Therapy. 2013;**15**(Suppl 3):S3. DOI: 10.1186/ar4175

[22] Manocha S, Lal D, Venkataraman S. Administration of h2 blockers in NSAID induced gastropathy in rats: Effect on histopathological changes in gastric, hepatic and renal tissues. Arquivos de Gastroenterologia. 2016;**53**(1):36-43. DOI: 10.1590/S0004-28032016000100008

[23] Molinari C, Morsanuto V, Ruga S, Stoppa I, Notte F, Farghali M, et al. Role of vitamin D3 and alginates in prevention of NSAID-dependent cellular injury. EC Gastroenterology and Digestive System. 2019;**6**:3, 211-223

[24] Pantziarka P, Sukhatme V, Bouche G, Meheus L, Sukhatme VP. Repurposing drugs in oncology (ReDO)-diclofenac as an anti-cancer agent. Ecancermedicalscience. 2016;**10**:610. DOI: 10.3332/ecancer.2016.610

[25] Gan TJ. Diclofenac: An update on its mechanism of action and safety profile. Current Medical Research and Opinion. 2010;**26**(7):1715-1731. DOI: 10.1185/03007995.2010.486301

[26] Rostom A, Dube C, Wells G, Tugwell P, Welch V, Jolicoeur E, et al. Prevention of NSAID-induced gastroduodenal ulcers. Cochrane Database of Systematic Reviews. 2002;**4**:CD002296

[27] Lau JY, Barkun A, Fan DM, Kuipers EJ, Yang YS, Chan FK. Challenges in the management of acute peptic ulcer bleeding. Lancet. 2013;**381**(9882):2033-2043. DOI: 10.1016/S0140-6736(13)60596-6

[28] Yamaguchi Y, Yoshikawa K. Cutaneous wound healing: An update. The Journal of Dermatology. 2001;**28**:521-523

[29] Leiman DA, Riff BP, Morgan S, Metz DC, Falk GW, French B, et al. Alginate therapy is effective treatment for GERD symptoms: A systematic review and meta-analysis. Diseases of the Esophagus. 2017;**30**(5):1-9. DOI: 10.1093/dote/dow020

[30] Sifrim D, Penagini R. Capping the gastric acid pocket to reduce postprandial acid gastroesophageal reflux. Clinical Gastroenterology and Hepatology. 2013;**11**:1592-1594. DOI: 10.1016/j.cgh.2013.06.008

[31] Lee KY, Mooney DJ. Alginate: Properties and biomedical applications. Progress in Polymer Science. 2012;**37**(1):106-126

[32] Matricardi P, Alhaique F, Coviello T, editors. Polysaccharide Hydrogels: Characterization and Biomedical Applications. Singapore: Pan Stanford Publishing Pte., Ltd; 2015. pp. 449-498

[33] Yuan YZ, Fang JY, Zou DW, Levinson N, Jenner B, Wilkinson J. Alginate-antacid (Gaviscon Double Action) chewable tablets reduce esophageal acid exposure in Chinese patients with gastroesophageal reflux disease and heartburn symptoms. Journal of Digestive Diseases. 2016;**17**(11):725-734. DOI: 10.1111/1751-2980.12406

[34] Tighe M, Afzal NA, Bevan A, Hayen A, Munro A, Beattie RM. Pharmacological treatment of children with gastro-oesophageal reflux. Cochrane Database of Systematic Reviews. 2014;**11**:CD008550. DOI: 10.1002/14651858.CD008550.pub2

[35] Hampson FC, Farndale A, Strugala V, Sykes J, Jolliffe IG, Dettmar PW. Alginate rafts and their characterisation. International Journal of Pharmaceutics. 2005;**294**(1-2):137-147

[36] Noguchi K, Kato K, Moriya T, Suzuki T, Saito M, Kikuchi T, et al. Analysis of cell damage in helicobacter pylori-associated gastritis. Pathology International. 2002;**52**(2):110-118

[37] Tran CD, Campbell MA, Kolev Y, Chamberlain S, Huynh HQ, Butler RN. Short-term zinc supplementation attenuates helicobacter felis-induced gastritis in the mouse. The Journal of Infection. 2005;**50**(5):417-424

[38] Kim JK, Oh SM, Kwon HS, Oh YS, Lim SS, Shin HK. Anti-inflammatory effect of roasted licorice extracts on lipopolysaccharide-induced inflammatory responses in murine macrophages. Biochemical and Biophysical Research Communications. 2006;**345**(3):1215-1223

[39] Alecci U, Bonina F, Bonina A, Rizza L, Inferrera S, Mannucci C, et al. Efficacy and safety of a natural remedy for the treatment of gastroesophageal reflux: A double-blinded randomized-controlled study. Evidence-based Complementary and Alternative Medicine. 2016;**2016**:2581461

[40] Bedemo A, Chandravanshi BS, Zewge F. Removal of trivalent chromium from aqueous solution using aluminum oxide hydroxide. Springerplus. 2016;**5**(1):1288. DOI: 10.1186/s40064-016-2983-x

[41] Bischoff-Ferrari HA. Optimal serum 25-hydroxyvitamin D levels for multiple health outcomes. Adv. Exp. Med. Biol. 2014;**810**:500-525

[42] Raman M, Milestone AN, Walters JR, Hart AL, Ghosh S. Vitamin D and gastrointestinal diseases: Inflammatory bowel disease and colorectal cancer. Therapeutic Advances in Gastroenterology. 2011;**4**(1):49-62. DOI: 10.1177/1756283X10377820

[43] Stumpf WE, Sar M, Reid FA, Tanaka Y, DeLuca HF. Target cells for 1,25-dihydroxyvitamin D3 in intestinal tract, stomach, kidney, skin, pituitary, and parathyroid. Science. 1979;**206**(4423):1188-1190

[44] Jones G, Strugnell SA, DeLuca HF. Current understanding

of the molecular actions of vitamin D. Physiological Reviews. 1998;**78**(4):1193-1231. DOI: 10.1152/physrev.1998.78.4.1193

[45] Thomas E, Wade A, Crawford G, Jenner B, Levinson N, Wilkinson J. Randomised clinical trial: Relief of upper gastrointestinal symptoms by an acid pocket-targeting alginate-antacid (Gaviscon Double Action)- a double- blind, placebo-controlled, pilot study in gastro-oesophageal reflux disease. Alimentary Pharmacology & Therapeutics. 2014;**39**(6):595-602. DOI: 10.1111/apt.12640

[46] Miyazaki Y, Shinomura Y, Tsutsui S, Yasunaga Y, Zushi S, Higashiyama S, et al. Oxidative stress increases gene expression of heparin-binding EGF-like growth factor and amphiregulin in cultured rat gastric epithelial cells. Biochemical and Biophysical Research Communications. 1996;**226**:542-546. DOI: 10.1006/bbrc.1996.1391

[47] Granger DN, Rutili G, McCord JM. Superoxide radicals in feline intestinal ischemia. Gastroenterology. 1981;**81**:22-29

[48] Itoh M, Guth PH. Role of oxygen-derived free radicals in hemorrhagic shock- induced gastric lesions in the rat. Gastroenterology. 1985;**88**:1162-1167

[49] Hirota M, Inoue M, Ando Y, Hirayama K, Morino Y, Sakamoto K, et al. Inhibition of stress-induced gastric injury in the rat by glutathione. Gastroenterology. 1989;**97**:853-859

Section 3

Technological Applications

Chapter 7

Importance of Alginate Bioink for 3D Bioprinting in Tissue Engineering and Regenerative Medicine

Sudipto Datta, Ranjit Barua and Jonali Das

Abstract

Among many bioinks used for extrusion 3D bioprinting, the most commonly used bioink is the polysaccharide alginate because of its various cellular-friendly property like gelation. Erratic degradation and cell-binding motifs are not present in alginate which are the limitations of alginate bioinks, which can be improved by blending various low concentrations of natural or artificial polymers. Here in this chapter, we will discuss the various important properties of the alginate which make it as the bioink for almost all bioprinting scaffold designs as well as how improve the cellular properties like its cell-material interaction by blending it with other polymer solutions.

Keywords: 3D bioprinting, alginate, bioink, hydrogel

1. Introduction

The main objective of three-dimensional (3D) printing is to print a living cell or to create a three-dimensional biomaterial's scaffold. This innovative technology allows the reproducible and also the automated fabrication of three-dimensional useful living tissues by depositing biomaterials layer by layer with an accurate positioning of cells. This method allows to make a three-dimensional object and an accurate as well as scalable geometries that are not suggested by any approaches like two-dimensional cell cultures [1].

The choice of applying these 3D functional living tissues comes from fundamental research [2]. Learning about the cell-biomaterial interface at the nanoscale stage is vital in accommodating flaws in tissues, nanoparticle-cell connections and organ defects [3], toxicological analysis or drug investigation [4], and transplantation in living objects [5]. Because of the rising complexity required for these tissues, 3D bioprinting is facing a lot of challenges in all of manufacturing areas. For example, the cell-encapsulated materials are commonly observable to chemical cross linkers for extended periods of time during storage prior to printing, which can harm the cells. At the time of deposition, the mechanical stress generated by the printing itself can result in damage and injury to cell functioning by cell shearing or extrusion [6]. The instant new printing tissue is fabricated, because of the small vascularity of printed material; limited nutrients are supplied in 3D construct [7].

Usually, the requirements for a suitable cell-containing dispensable biomaterial or bioink are generally biocompatibility, exhaustive, biomimicry, printability, and essential mechanical properties. This is the main cause for the huge number of the manufacturers of commercially accessible 3D bioprinters—particularly extrusion-based 3D bioprinter, where hydrogel bioinks are recommended [8]. Particularly, hydrogels are unquestionably the most comprehensive biomaterials applied as cell matrix in bioinks because they can be engaged as cell matrix and be modified to replace or mimic local tissue [9]. The physical and chemical characteristics of the hydrogels will verify the performance of the cells. Normally hydrogels are like as jelly-type materials, where the liquid component is water. Actually, hydrogels are just like water by weight, but practically any flow will not occur in the steady state because of the three-dimensional cross-linked polymer network inside the fluid, which provides them unique properties comparable to those of living tissues. Due to their different biocompatibility and printability, various hydrogels that support cell growth are associated with bioink fabrication, i.e., gelatin, agarose, polyethylene glycol (PEG)-diacrylate, and alginate that are commonly used as bioinks. While alginate is an anionic polysaccharide derived from brown seaweed and generally consists of two polymer blocks, (1-4)-linked β-D-mannuronate (M) and its C-5 epimer α-L-guluronate (G) residues, basically all are covalently linked. The main elements in the alginic acid polymer chain are the carboxylic acid group which allows cross-linking. This converts alginate from its liquid state to a semisolid gel state. Sodium alginate is mostly used as bioink in tissue engineering and cell culture because of biocompatibility, low-cost, and fast gelation. In **Figure 1**, the presence of calcium ions and ionic interactions between Ca^{2+} and COO^{-} occur, and cross-linking of alginate polymers results.

Ionic cross-linking is a method where cells cause minimum damage. The cross-linking process happens moderately rapidly. Alginate has structural similarity to natural extracellular matrices that is why it has been applied widely in various biomedical applications as well as in the delivery of bioactive agents and wound healing. For cell encapsulation, alginate hydrogels are generally applied. The whole procedure is prepared by mixing cells in alginate solution, and after the mixing process, the alginate-cell mixture drops into a bath of calcium chloride solution. But in low concentrations (1–2%), due to low viscosity, the alginate solution is not printable. For increasing the viscosity, other materials like methylcellulose or gelatin can be mixed with alginate for preparing the printability. The structural correspondence of alginate to extracellular matrices creates a perfect biomaterial. Matrix stiffness is a functional determinant of stem cell differentiation, and alginate makes a potential material to manage stem cell growth. Alginate helps support the cell growth and also has a high versatility, extending to both in vivo and in vitro differentiation. For 3D bioprinting applications, for example, extrusion printing needs quick gelation. In this case alginate proposes high gelation procedures when combined with a

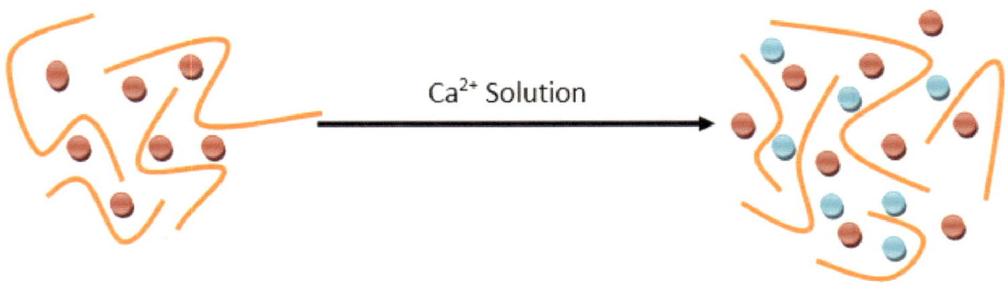

Figure 1.
Cross-linking process of alginate.

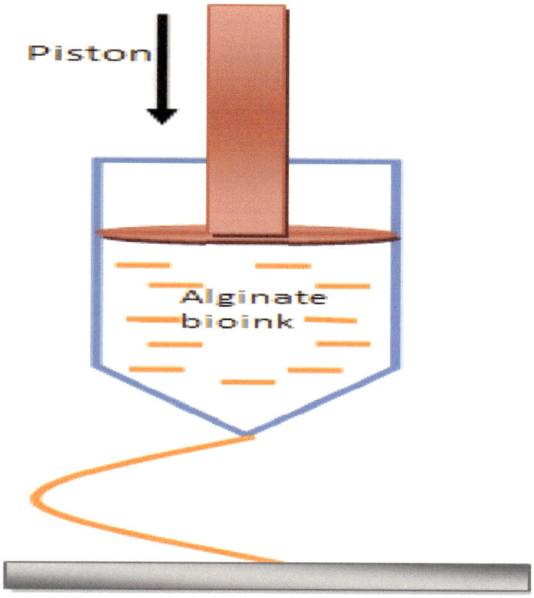

Figure 2.
Extrusion-based 3D bioprinting process.

multivalent cation, permitting gels to build up and deposit at constant temperature. It is also applied to encapsulate cells. This allows it to be an effective tool in varying the release rate of drug and growth factor delivery. While alginate degradation rate can be somewhat controlled by altering the MW of the alginate, it is still slow and difficult to control. The stiffness and composition properties of alginate bioink can be tuned to direct the differentiation of stem cells. Sodium alginate is available naturally which is biodegradable, non-immunogenic linear, and nontoxic polysaccharide polymer; it consists of mannuronic and guluronic acids [10]. The cost is also low being a marine material which can be extracted from the brown algae cell walls, forming hydrogel in certain conditions. Because of these advantages, bioengineers and material scientists use alginate for the preparation of bioinks in tissue engineering and regenerative medicines. The tissue fabrication by 3D bioprinting [11] and sodium alginate applications and properties [12] is currently separately reviewed. In this study we discussed the applications of alginate (**Figure 2**) in 3D bioprinting and blending alginate with other polymers to improve the biomaterial interaction of the cells attached to it [13].

2. Application of alginate

The requirement for alginate-based biomaterials in drug delivery and tissue engineering is huge. As stem cells play a progressively more major function in the area of regenerative medicine [14, 15], the arrangement and relation between alginate-based materials and stem cells have been exclusively emphasized. Investigated by in vitro implantation and in vitro cytotoxicity assay, alginate-based scaffolds and microcapsules have shown minimum or minor cytotoxicity [16, 17]. These in vitro results recommended tunable connections between the bio-composites and the multiple platelet releasate-derived bioagents for improving hematoma-like fracture repair. Also, a simple invasive performance for in situ remedial of the implant structures through injection was established in rat tail vertebrae applying microcomputed tomography. These results confirmed that alginate-based scaffolds were capable of degrading, permitted the vascularization, and obtained minimum inflammatory responses after transplantation. Consequently, alginate-based scaffolds can present suitable characteristics as probable cell and drug carriers for tissue regeneration. The next sections explain the clinical and preclinical analysis of alginate-based biomaterials and applications.

2.1 3D bioprinting

Sodium alginate which is also known as sodium alginate or algin is a naturally extracted less costly polymer from the brown algae cell walls which have intracellular spaces [10]. Alginate is composed of (1-4)-linked β-D-mannuronic (M) and α-L-guluronic acids (G). Alginate is a polyanionic linear block copolymer made of longer M or G blocks, separated by MG regions. Sodium alginate is a kind of polysaccharide which is charged negatively because it is known that materials which are positively charged produce inflammatory response; this allows the biopolymer to support high biocompatibility and cell growth. G blocks enhance the gel structure and M and MG blocks enhance the elasticity, though a high quantity of M blocks could be the reason of immunogenicity [18]. In alginate matrix, with the help of capillary forces, water and other molecules can be trapped. This feature makes alginate hydrogel suitable for bioink designs. The cell density within the bioink will be very high, whereas the shear stress through the extrusion process decreases the cell viability (80–90%). In the case of inkjet bioprinting, the bioinks have lower cell densities ($<16 \times 106$ cells/mL) and are less viscous (<10 mPa s). This technique suggests 90% cell viabilities but, in laser-assisted bioprinting, needs bioinks with viscosities of 1 and 300 mPa s and also requires medium cell densities (108 cells/mL). In this method, cell viability is very high (>95%). The alginate-based bioink viscosity rests on the alginate molecular weight, alginate concentration, density of cells, and cell phenotype. These are the variables that scientist must consider to optimize the viscosity of the alginate-based bioinks. An additional significant rheological characteristic of aqueous alginate solutions is the shear-thinning, where the shear rate increases while decreasing the viscosity. The viscosity also depends on the performed printing temperature; when the temperature increases, the viscosity gradually decreases. In comparison with other polymers, alginate is convincingly easy to handle and to print and is easy to extrude (printing) while defending the encapsulated cells. Even if it is also a non-cell-adhesive [12], in case of cell encapsulation, alginate is currently one of the most applied biomaterials. After the printing performance, the hydrogel should degrade suitably, allowing the cells to make their specific extra cellular matrix (ECM). The alginate also generates durable insistent cell-laden hydrogels; however oxidation can be performed by slow degradation, for example, sodium peroxide [11]. The main issue of alginate for using it as a biomaterial in bioprinting is slow degradation rate. The release of the hydrogels through the bioprinter nozzle in bioprinting (extrusion) limits the usage to low weight of alginate, which has a major role in the application of reduced mechanical properties. Though the alginate mechanical and structural characteristics are needed for all printed tissue, the biomimicry characteristics required in every instance can be changed by combining new biomaterials in the scaffold or by applying different types of hydrogel fabrication technique. For example, CELLINK is a commercial bioink which is already available for bioprinting; it combines with alginate hydrogel and nanocellulose and presents fast cross-linking and shear-thinning properties; this bioink is appreciated for soft tissue engineering for bioprinting [8]. The formation of blood vessel-like channels is able to transport different materials like nutrients and oxygen via the bioprinted material, which is needed in order to print organs or tissues. To succeed in this aim, Zhang et al. [19] made vessel-like printable microfluidic channels where a coaxial nozzle strategy is used for transporting the nutrient into printed material, and the printer was pressure-assisted bioprinter and the coaxial needle was applied for printing the hollow alginate filaments that contain cartilage progenitor cells. In the same way, a triaxial nozzle assembly was used to fabricate biocompatible cartilage-like tissues containing tubular channels, where the alginate was encapsulated by cartilage progenitor cells, which is the main element of the bioink. Hydrogels of sodium alginate having high strength and having inner microchannels were found out by Gao et al. [20]. Also, constructs like perfusable vascular-like constructs were also obtained through coaxial multilayered nozzle along with the concentric extrusion channel by 3D printing in one step [21] by mixing 4-arm poly(ethylene glycol)-tetra-acrylate (PEGTA) and gelatin methacryloyl (GelMA) with the sodium alginate. Calcium ions were used to cross-link the alginate, and photo-cross-linking was used for covalent cross-linking for PEGTA and GelMA for setting the rheological and mechanical properties that was reported in this work. Also in another study, Christensen et al. [12] printed vascular structures along with bifurcations (vertical and horizontal) in alginate and fibroblast of mouse bioinks. Blending alginate with other polymers (honey, gelatin) [22], amino acids like polyglutamic acid and poly-L-lysine [13, 23], and some drugs like N-acetylcysteine (NAC) [24] was studied for improving the erratic degradation, cell-material interaction, cell viability, etc. The printer (inkjet) used $CaCl_2$ cross-linking agent supporting material for cross-linking the alginate bioink. To back up the buoyant force in the regions overhanging in both vertical and horizontal printing and also supporting the regions spanning in the horizontal printing, their modified solution was used. Blending alginate with other polymers (honey, gelatin) [22], amino acids like (polyglutamic acid and poly-L-lysine) [13, 23], and some drugs like N-acetylcysteine (NAC) [24] was studied for improving the erratic degradation, cell-material interaction, cell viability, etc. Jia et al. [6] in their study showed the controlled degradation of oxidized alginate in 3D bioprinting.

Varying biodegradability of solution of sodium alginate along with human adipose stem cells was printed with accurate definition. These kinds of bioinks have the capacity to modulate proliferation and stem cell spreading and withstand uniform cell suspension but are imperfect in the case of stem cell diffusion. Wu et al. [25] showed the procedure of slow degradation of the alginate by tissue incubation in a sodium citrate medium. The sodium citrate amount helped the optimization of the alginate degradation time. Chung et al. [18] improved the printing resolution and printability of pre-crosslinked printed constructs by adding alginate with gelatin, keeping the mechanical property and the growth of cells, and keeping pore diameter constant. In **Figure 3** the procedure of alginate cross-linking with the added cells is shown.

2.2 Wound healing

Alginate has been used for dressing of the wounds due to its of good conformability, absorptivity, and mild antiseptic properties coupled with biodegradability and nontoxicity and optimal water vapor transmission rate. Alginate-based products like electrospun mat hydrogels and sponges in dressing of wounds are very good substrates for healing of wounds, which include gel-foaming capability as soon as the absorption of the wound exudates and hemostatic capabilities [26]. It is already been mentioned that dressing wounds with alginate improves healing of wounds through monocyte stimulation to harvest higher cytokine levels like tumor necrosis factor-α and interleukin-6 [27]. Near the wound locations, cytokine production creates pro-inflammatory factors that are helpful for wound healing. Because of the existence of endotoxin in the alginate, a huge level of bioactivity

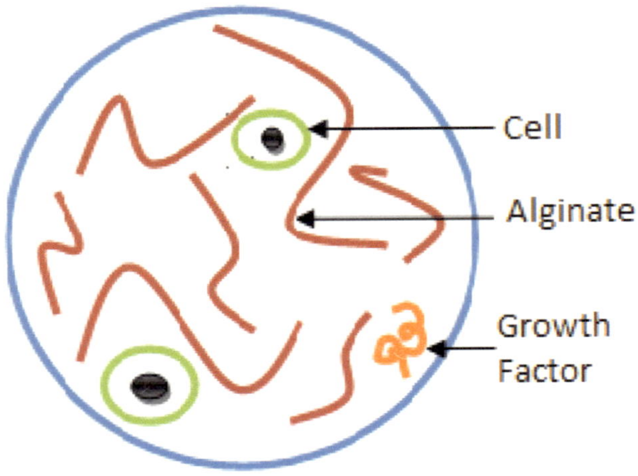

Figure 3.
Alginate with cell cross-linking process.

is present in these dressings. In situ-forming wound dressing hydrogel can be produced by oxidized alginate and gelatin in low borax concentration as shown by Balakrishnan and Jayakrishnan [28]. The homeostatic gelatin effect is present in the mixed matrix and wound healing property of alginate, and the antiseptic borax property makes alginate the appropriate wound dressing material. Tissue-engineered cartilage requirement is immense and has a huge clinical importance. The main causes of disability of the articular cartilage are degenerative and traumatic lesions [29]. Nearly 100 million Chinese people suffer from osteoarthritis. Because of this reason, regeneration and repair of the cartilage have huge impact. The pros of the cartilage repair injectable therapies are that implant within the defect is not only maintained, but it also allows quick bearing of weight because of strength and stiffness which is attained quickly [30, 31]. For bringing close the mechanical properties of the native tissues with the scaffolds, the alginate physical properties are matched with the articular cartilage. Ge and solid alginate injectable hydrogel microspheres are used for cartilage regeneration. Many researchers have studied the growth factor in tissue engineering by using alginate hydrogels and alginate-based microsphere combinations [32, 33]. In one study the demonstration of immobilization of the positive effect of RGD to an alginate porous scaffold for endorsing TGF-β-induced human MSC differentiation is shown [34]. Bian et al. studied the co-encapsulation of the TGF-β including the microsphere of the alginate with the human MSCs in the hyaluronic acid (HA) hydrogels with respect to the design of the constructs implantable for the cartilage repair [35]. The immobilized RGD peptide facilitated the cell-matrix interaction which is proven to be an important feature for the microenvironment of the cells, allowing good cell availability for the chondrogenic-inducing molecule TGF-β. TGF-β-laden alginate microspheres in combination with alginate hydrogels forms a compound carrier which may retain TGF-β bioactivity in the construct and encourages hondrogenesis of MSCs when inserted. The animal experiment displayed that chondrocytes planted into the microsphere scaffold lived habitually in SCID mice and cartilage-like constructions were created after 4 weeks of imbedding.

2.3 Drug delivery

In the past years, drug delivery carriers draw huge interest because of large biomacromolecules like genes and proteins as well as low-molecule weight drugs which can be delivered in a targeted or a localized manner [36, 37]. Because of its biodegradable and biocompatible nature, alginate is used as a carrier for encapsulating and immobilizing drugs, cells, proteins, and bioactive molecules [38, 39]. Currently, alginate-based carriers like colloidal particles, polyelectrolyte, and hydrogels are under examination; few of them are practically used. Many researchers have examined the alginate-based hydrogel blends, microspheres, and porous scaffolds for precise drug delivery in various tissue engineering fields [40, 41]. Hollow microsphere of alginate-based hollow microsphere has huge applications as drug delivery carrier, micro-reactor, and biosensor [42]. The construction of the hollow microcapsules can be created by successive self-assembly of positively and negatively charged polyelectrolytes by layer-by-layer (LbL) technique. The alginate microcapsule is studied well with respect to precise releasing and loading parameters. The attempt to fabricate microcapsule biopolymer has been made by dropping alginate/chitosan in a decomposable colloid particle after removal of its core is done in an appropriate pathway. For the production of hollow microcapsule, chitosan and alginate are interchangeably deposited in $CaCO_3$ with electrostatic biocompatibility [43]. The chitosan/alginate microcapsule functionalities and properties can be preciously adjusted by changing the microcapsule composition, exterior stimuli introduction, and thickness. Immersing alginate microcapsule in various pH solutions helps in the degradation of the microcapsules which also determines the material role and encapsulation layers for keeping microcapsule stability in various pH conditions. The addition of PEG to the microcapsule allows protection against acidic conditions, whereas the coating layer number only affects the swelling properties, not the microcapsule Young's modulus which was revealed by Wong's study [9]. For surface micro-patternings and microarray systems, 3D platform alginate hydrogels are used. For in situ gelation, a few aliquots of solution of gelatin were trapped selectively on hydrophilic area by a process called dipping process. Cells with various adhesion properties were captured by gel pattern alginate on the hydrogel structures.

Various CYP450 enzymes like vascular endothelial growth factor (VEGF) and β1-integrin upregulation showed that the stage gave many in vitro conditions that result in allowing cells in their natural phenotypes.

2.4 Bone regeneration

For the reconstructive surgery, bone regeneration is an important challenge. It occurs due to tumor removal and trauma. To repair the bone, a good initiative is to induce osteogenesis in situ. To complete this process, one method is by using stem cell differentiation to form bone tissue and then seeding them in an injectable scaffold [44, 45]. As of now there are numerous investigations and studies on alginate-based injectable scaffolds for the bone regeneration. By using MSCs and alginate scaffolds, satisfactory bone tissue formation was noticed [46, 47]. For this reason the application of alginate for gel tissue generation is commonly used which displays angiogenic and osteogenic properties. Many researchers showed bone regeneration by means of injectable constructs by joining microspheres or alginate-based hydrogels that were combined with interchangeable ASCs or MSCs [48]. These studies demonstrated the potential of bone morphogenetic protein (BMP) and TGF-β delivery to induce osteogenic differentiation to mature osteocytes from MSCs and ASCs. Kolambkar et al. presented a growth factor hybrid system of delivery that comprises of a nanofiber mesh tube *which is electrospun* for directing regeneration of bone along with alginate hydrogel peptide modified in the tube for fixed recombination BMP-2 (rhBMP-2) release [49]. The discharge of fixed transport of rhBMP-2 through alginate hydrogel was important for significant regeneration to take place. The mixed technology can be used clinically for the regeneration of bone in cases as huge bone defect and nonunion fractures.

3. Conclusions

The naturally available biopolymer alginate is cheaper which forms hydrogel by cross-linking with various salts like $BaCl_2$, $CaCl_2$, and $ZnCl_2$ which showed good biocompatibility and printability.

This is broadly applied for cartilage, bone, and vascular tissue printing. Few drawbacks of alginate are slow degradation and poor cell adhesion; in many research, it is shown that alginate has poor cell differentiation and cell proliferation, and for this reason, it is used as a blend with other polymers. To improve these limitations, blending alginate with other polymers like honey, gelatin, and Arg-Gly-Asp adhesions is done. Furthermore, for faster normal degradation in regenerative medicine, oxidized alginate and/or sodium citrate is found to be useful. The combination of 3D printing alginate for cartilage and electrospinning is used positively in various tissue engineering fields. Furthermore, mixing alginate with biopolymers like polycaprolactone and nanocellulose has shown positive results. In bioprinting using coaxial or triaxial nozzles is found out to be promising and provided brilliant results. To improve the mechanical properties of the alginate-based structures used in bone tissue engineering, mixing alginate with other polymers like bio-silica, polyphosphate, polycaprolactone hydroxyapatite, and gelatin is found to produce an excellent result. We think this review will allow researchers to investigate more advanced and improved bioink for 3D printing and also help to invent suitable and more appropriate bioink for various tissue engineering applications

Author details

Sudipto Datta[1*], Ranjit Barua[1] and Jonali Das[2]

1 Centre for Healthcare Science and Technology, Indian Institute of Engineering Science and Technology Shibpur, Howrah, W.B., India

2 Department of Chemistry, Raja Peary Mohan Collage, Calcutta University, Uttarpara, W.B., India

*Address all correspondence to: dattadip440v@gmail.com

References

[1] Devillard R, Pagès E, Correa MM, Kériquel V, Rémy M, Kalisky J, et al. Cell patterning by laser-assisted bioprinting. Methods in Cell Biology. 2014;**119**:159-174

[2] Kang HW, Lee SJ, Ko IK, Kengla C, Yoo JJ, Atala A. A 3D bioprinting system to produce human-scale tissue constructs with structural integrity. Nature Biotechnology. 2016;**34**:312-319

[3] Miller JS. The billion cell construct: Will three-dimensional printing get us there? PLoS Biology. 2014;**12**:e1001882

[4] Murphy SV, Atala A. 3D bioprinting of tissues and organs. Nature Biotechnology. 2014;**32**:773-785

[5] Kulseng B, Skjåk-Braek G, Ryan L, Andersson A, King A, Faxvaag A, et al. Transplantation of alginate microcapsules: Generation of antibodies against alginates and encapsulated porcine islet-like cell clusters. Transplantation. 1999;**67**:978-984

[6] Jia J, Richards DJ, Pollard S, Tan Y, Rodriguez J, Visconti RP, et al. Engineering alginate as bioink for bioprinting. Acta Biomaterialia. 2014;**10**:4323-4331

[7] Boontheekul T, Kong H-J, Mooney DJ. Controlling alginate gel degradation utilizing partial oxidation and bimodal molecular weight distribution. Biomaterials. 2005;**26**:2455-2465

[8] Kong HJ, Kaigler D, Kim K, Mooney DJ. Controlling rigidity and degradation of alginate hydrogels via molecular weight distribution. Biomacromolecules. 2004;**5**:1720-1727

[9] Wong TY, Preston LA, Schiller NL. ALGINATE LYASE: Review of major sources and enzyme characteristics, structure-function analysis, biological roles, and applications. Annual Review of Microbiology. 2000;**54**:289-340

[10] Yu Y, Zhang Y, Martin JA, Ozbolat IT. Evaluation of cell viability and functionality in vessel-like bioprintable cell-laden tubular channels. Journal of Biomechanical Engineering. 2013;**135**:91011

[11] Jia W, Gungor-Ozkerim PS, Zhang YS, Yue K, Zhu K, Liu W, et al. Direct 3D bioprinting of perfusable vascular constructs using a blend bioink. Biomaterials. 2016;**106**:58-68

[12] Christensen K, Xu C, Chai W, Zhang Z, Fu J, Huang Y. Freeform inkjet printing of cellular structures with bifurcations. Biotechnology and Bioengineering. 2015;**112**:1047-1055

[13] Datta S, Barua R, Sarkar R, Barui A, Roy Chowdhury A, Datta P. Design and development of alginate: Poly-l-lysine scaffolds by 3D bio printing and studying their mechanical, structural and cell viability. In: IOP Conference Series: Materials Science and Engineering. 2018

[14] Tan H, Marra KG. Injectable, biodegradable hydrogels for tissue engineering applications. Materials. 2010;**3**:1746-1767

[15] Tememoff JS, Mikos AG. Injectable biodegradable materials for orthopedic tissue engineering. Biomaterials. 2000;**21**:2405-2412

[16] Li X, Chen S, Zhang B, Li M, Diao K, Zhang Z, et al. *In situ* injectable nano-composite hydrogel composed of curcumin, N,O-carboxymethyl chitosan and oxidized alginate for wound healing application. International Journal of Pharmaceutics. 2012;**437**:110-119

[17] Hooper SJ, Percival SL, Hill KE, Thomas DW, Hayes AJ, Williams DW.

The visualisation and speed of kill of wound isolates on a silver alginate dressing. International Wound Journal. 2012;**9**:633-642

[18] Chung JHY, Naficy S, Yue Z, Kapsa R, Quigley A, Moulton SE, et al. Bio-ink properties and printability for extrusion printing living cells. Biomaterials Science. 2013;**1**:763-773

[19] Zhang Y, Yu Y, Chen H, Ozbolat IT. Characterization of printable cellular micro-fluidic channels for tissue engineering. Biofabrication. 2013;**5**:025004

[20] Gao Q, He Y, Fu J-Z, Liu A, Ma L. Coaxial nozzle-assisted 3D bioprinting with built-in microchannels for nutrients delivery. Biomaterials. 2015;**61**:203-215

[21] Armstrong JPK, Burke M, Carter BM, Davis SA, Perriman AW. 3D bioprinting using a templated porous bioink. Advanced Healthcare Materials. 2016;**5**:1724-1730

[22] Datta S, Sarkar R, Vyas V, Bhutoria S, Barui A, Roy Chowdhury A, et al. Alginate-honey bioinks with improved cell responses for applications as bioprinted tissue engineered constructs. Journal of Materials Research. 2018;**33**(14):2029-2039

[23] Datta S, Das A, Sasmal P, Bhutoria S, Roy Chowdhury A, Datta P. Alginate-poly (amino acid) extrusion printed scaffolds for tissueengineering applications. International Journal of Polymeric Materials and Polymeric Biomaterials. 2018;**69**(2):1-9

[24] Datta S, Das A, Roy Chowdhury A, Datta P. Bioink formulations to ameliorate bioprinting-induced loss of cellular viability. Biointerphases. 2019;**14**(5):051006

[25] Wu Z, Su X, Xu Y, Kong B, Sun W, Mi S. Bioprinting three-dimensional cell-laden tissue constructs with controllable degradation. Scientific Reports. 2016;**6**:24474

[26] Abbah SA, Liu J, Lam RW, Goh JC, Wong HK. *In vitro* bioactivity of rhBMP-2 delivered with novel polyelectrolyte complexation shells assembled on an alginate microbead core template. Journal of Controlled Release. 2012;**162**:364-372

[27] Huang SH, Hsueh HJ, Jiang YL. Light-addressable electrodeposition of cell-encapsulated alginate hydrogels for a cellular microarray using a digital micromirror device. Biomicrofluidics. 2011;**5**:34109:1-34109:10

[28] Balakrishnan B, Jayakrishnan A. Self-cross-linking biopolymers as injectable *in situ* forming biodegradable scaffolds. Biomaterials. 2005;**26**:3941-3951

[29] Sugaya S, Kakegawa S, Fukushima S, Yamada M, Seki M. Micropatterning of hydrogels on locally hydrophilized regions on PDMS by stepwise solution dipping and *in situ* gelation. Langmuir. 2012;**28**:14073-14080

[30] Cao Y, Shen XC, Chen Y, Guo J, Chen Q, Jiang XQ. pH-induced self-assembly and capsules of sodium alginate. Biomacromolecules. 2005;**6**:2189-2196

[31] Gombotz WR, Wee SF. Protein release from alginate matrices. Advanced Drug Delivery Reviews. 1998;**31**:267-285

[32] Folkman J, Hochberg M. Self-regulation of growth in three dimensions. The Journal of Experimental Medicine. 1973;**138**:745-753

[33] Neufurth M, Wang X, Schröder HC, Feng Q, Diehl-Seifert B, Ziebart T, et al. Engineering a morphogenetically active hydrogel for bioprinting of bioartificial

tissue derived from human osteoblast-like SaOS-2 cells. Biomaterials. 2014;**35**:8810-8819

[34] Daly AC, Cunniffe GM, Sathy BN, Jeon O, Alsberg E, Kelly DJ. 3D bioprinting of developmentally inspired templates for whole bone organ engineering. Advanced Healthcare Materials. 2016 Sep;**5**(18):2353-2362. DOI: 10.1002/adhm.201600182. [Epub Jun 9 2016]

[35] Bian L, Zhai DY, Tous E, Rai R, Mauck RL, Burdick JA. Enhanced MSC chondrogenesis following delivery of TGF-β3 from alginate microspheres within hyaluronic acid hydrogels *in vitro* and *in vitro*. Biomaterials. 2011;**32**:6425-6434

[36] Gruene M, Pflaum M, Deiwick A, Koch L, Schlie S, Unger C, et al. Adipogenic differentiation of laser-printed 3D tissue grafts consisting of human adipose-derived stem cells. Biofabrication. 2011;**3**(1):005-015

[37] Ozbolat IT, Hospodiuk M. Current advances and future perspectives in extrusion-based bioprinting. Biomaterials. 2016;**76**:321-343

[38] Yanez M, Rincon J, Dones A, De Maria C, Gonzales R, Boland T. *In Vivo* assessment of printed microvasculature in a bilayer skin graft to treat full-thickness wounds. Tissue Engineering Part A. 2015;**21**(1-2):224-233

[39] Gudapati H, Yan J, Huang Y, Chrisey DB. Alginate gelation-induced cell death during laser-assisted cell printing. Biofabrication. 2014;**6**(3):022-035

[40] Cui X, Boland T. Human microvasculature fabrication using thermal inkjet printing technology. Biomaterials. 2009;**30**(31):6221-6227

[41] Freier T, Koh HS, Kazazian K, Shoichet MS. Controlling cell adhesion and degradation of chitosan films by N-acetylation. Biomaterials. 2005;**26**(29):5872-5878

[42] Tomei AA, Manzoli V, Fraker CV, Giraldo J, Velluto D, Najjar M, et al. Device design and materials optimization of conformal coating for islets of Langerhans. National Academy of Sciences. 2014;**111**(29): 10514-10519

[43] Holland NB, Qiu Y, Ruegsegger M, Marchant RE. Biomimetic engineering of non-adhesive glycocalyx-like surfaces using oligosaccharide surfactant polymers. Nature. 1998;**392**(6678):799-801

[44] Yahia LH. History and applications of hydrogels. Journal of Biomedical Science. 2015;**4**(2):1-23

[45] Chimene D, Lennox KK, Kaunas RR, Gaharwar AR. Advanced bioinks for 3D printing: A materials science perspective. Annals of Biomedical Engineering. 2016;**44**(6):2090-2102

[46] Cornelissen DJ, Faulkner-Jones A, Shu W. Current developments in 3D bioprinting for tissue engineering. Current Opinion in Biomedical Engineering. 2017;**2**:76-82

[47] Alsberg E, Anderson KW, Albeiruti A, Rowley JA, Mooney DJ. Engineering growing tissues. National Academy of Sciences. 2002;**99**(19):12025-12030

[48] Geng L, Feng W, Hutmacher DW, San Wong Y, Tong Loh H, Fuh JYH. Direct writing of chitosan scaffolds using a robotic system. Rapid Prototyping Journal. 2005;**11**(2):90-97

[49] Kolambkar YM, Dupont KM, Boerckel JD, Huebsch N, Mooney DJ, Hutmacher DW, et al. An alginate-based hybrid system for growth factor delivery in the functional repair of large bone defects. Biomaterials. 2011;**32**:65-74

Chapter 8

Application of Artificial Intelligence in Modern Healthcare System

Sudipto Datta, Ranjit Barua and Jonali Das

Abstract

Artificial intelligence (AI) has the potential of detecting significant interactions in a dataset and also it is widely used in several clinical conditions to expect the results, treat, and diagnose. Artificial intelligence (AI) is being used or trialed for a variety of healthcare and research purposes, including detection of disease, management of chronic conditions, delivery of health services, and drug discovery. In this chapter, we will discuss the application of artificial intelligence (AI) in modern healthcare system and the challenges of this system in detail. Different types of artificial intelligence devices are described in this chapter with the help of working mechanism discussion. Alginate, a naturally available polymer found in the cell wall of the brown algae, is used in tissue engineering because of its biocompatibility, low cost, and easy gelation. It is composed of α-L-guluronic and β-D-manuronic acid. To improve the cell-material interaction and erratic degradation, alginate is blended with other polymers. Here, we discuss the relationship of artificial intelligence with alginate in tissue engineering fields.

Keywords: artificial intelligence (AI), machine learning (ML), natural language processing (NLP), medical imaging, SVM

1. Introduction

Artificial intelligence (AI) technique is the most effective technology used in the modern healthcare area. The rapidly growing accessibility of healthcare medical data and also the advances of big data diagnostic techniques has completed the potential of the current successful uses of artificial intelligence (AI) in healthcare system. With the help of important medical questions, potential artificial intelligence (AI) techniques can disengage healthcare-appropriate information secreted in the huge quantity of data, which can maintain healthcare decision-making. Modern healthcare technology in various medical areas has spread to the several pioneering startups in the world, which helps people in healthier and longer lives. The advances have initially been determined by the beginning of mobility and software, permitting the health sector to digitize several of the pen- and paper-based processes and operations that are presently held up service release. Nowadays, computer software has become far more intelligent and autonomous. These new abilities are discussed under the same cover of machine learning (ML) and artificial intelligence (AI), which are accelerating the tempo of improvement in healthcare. The applications

IntechOpen

of machine learning (ML) and artificial intelligence (AI) in healthcare region have allowed the area to employ some of its major challenges in particular domains like drug discovery, personal genetics, and disease identification and management. Every time an innovative technical tool comes into the healthcare system, it also faces several challenges. Most of the common issues of artificial intelligence (AI) technique in healthcare system are regulatory compliance requirements, patient and provider adoption, and also lack of data exchange. The Artificial intelligence (AI) has moved from all of these concerns, reducing the areas in which it can accomplish something. The purpose of artificial intelligence (AI) and machine learning (ML) in healthcare system is redesigning the industry and creating what was once impracticable into a real truth. For artificial intelligence (AI)/machine learning (ML) to take its place in the healthcare system, sustained access to appropriate data is necessary to succeed. Artificial intelligence (AI) can be used to analyze and identify patterns in large and complex datasets faster and more precisely than has previously been possible. It can also be used to search the scientific literature for relevant studies and to combine different kinds of data, for example, to aid drug discovery. Artificial intelligence (AI) health apps have the potential to empower people to evaluate their own symptoms and care for themselves when possible. Artificial intelligence (AI) systems that aim to support people with chronic health conditions or disabilities could increase people's sense of dignity, independence, and quality of life, and enable people who may otherwise have been admitted to care institutions to stay at home for longer. Artificial intelligence (AI) depends on digital data, so inconsistencies in the availability and quality of data restrict the potential of artificial intelligence (AI). Also, significant computing power is required for the analysis of large and complex datasets. Clinical practice often involves complex judgments and abilities that artificial intelligence (AI) currently is unable to replicate, such as appropriate knowledge and the ability to read social cues. With the help of machine learning process, structured data like genetic data, electro physical data (EP), and imaging data are properly investigated. Machine learning makes the information analytical algorithms to extract characteristics from the input data. Input data generally in machine learning algorithms involve with patient's natures as well as the intermittently apprehension healing effects. A patient's nature generally includes bottom line data, such as gender, disease history, age, gene expressions, electrophysiological data (EP) test, analytical imaging, idea test results, and medicinal symptoms. Support vector machine was also applied in cancer diagnosis. Even supposing complicated data, machine learning represents the support for artificial intelligence (AI). At this moment in time, an innovative advancement is happening in the subfield of neural networks. This has created notable interest in various domains of healthcare science, in addition to drug analysis and also the area of public health. Deep neural networks can implement in addition to the most exceptional human clinicians in specific diagnostic tasks. Also, artificial intelligence techniques are already promising in healthcare-based apps, which can be performed by any network machine like modern smart mobile phone. Artificial intelligence has the ability to address imperative health challenges, but it is limited due to the unavailability of good health data. Employing artificial intelligence (AI) involves some ethical issues including the probable for artificial intelligence (AI) to make mistaken assessments and then the question of responsibility occurs.

2. Artificial intelligence (AI) devices

Basically, artificial intelligence (AI) devices are categorized by two main types: the first one is machine learning (ML) category [1], which generally analyses the structured data, for example, electrophysiological data (EP), genetic data, and imaging data. For healthcare applications, the machine learning (ML) processes try to gather patients' individuality or understand the possibility of the disease effects [2]. The second type of artificial intelligence (AI) device is the natural language processing (NLP) technique [3], which can take out the information from free or unstructured data such as medical observations or health journals to enhance structured health check data. The natural language processing (NLP) processes objects at revolving contents toward the machine-understandable structured records and can then be considered by machine learning (ML) procedures [4]. **Figure 1** explains the road plan from medical data making, during natural language processing (NLP) data improvement and machine learning (ML) data investigation, to medical judgment creating. In this figure, the road plan starts and ends with medical activities. As dominant as artificial intelligence (AI) procedures, they can be inspired by medical/healthcare troubles and also be practical to help out the medical performance at the end.

2.1 Machine learning (ML) processes

Machine learning (ML) builds the data investigative algorithms to extort characteristics from the data. Inputs to machine learning (ML) algorithms consist of patient 'characters' and occasionally therapeutic effects of concern. A patient's characters generally contain bottom line data, for example, gender, age, disease history, and also disease explicit data, for instance, gene expressions, analytical imaging, electrophysiological data (EP) test, objective test results, medication, and medical symptoms. In addition to the attributes of the patients medical results are frequently composed for medical investigation. These contain syndrome pointers, patients' endurance periods, and quantitative syndrome stages such as the size of tumor. Here j^{th} characteristic of the ith numbers of patient is denoted by P_{ij} and Q_i is representing the effect of concern. Regarding whether to integrate the results, machine learning (ML) algorithms can also be separated into two main types: supervised learning and unsupervised learning. One more type is also available

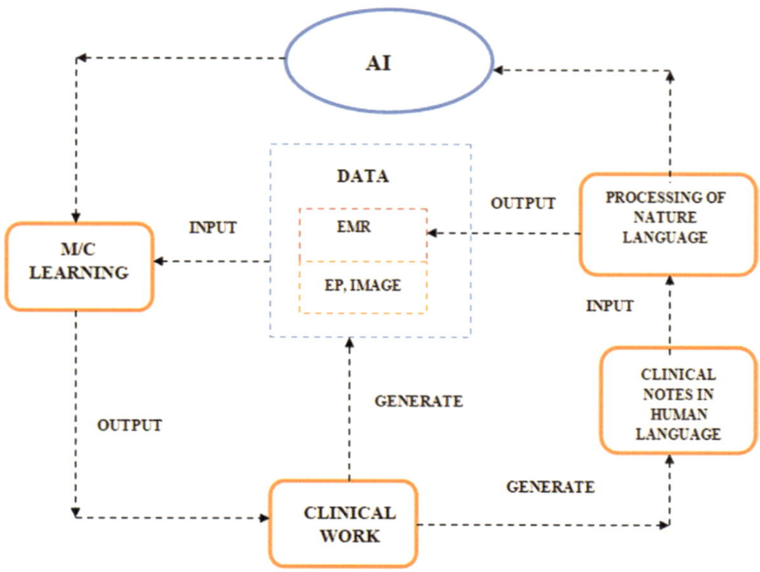

Figure 1.
The road plan from generation of medical data, during natural language processing (NLP) data improvement and machine learning (ML) data investigation.

named as semisupervised learning. **Figure 2** represents all these three types of learning procedures. Unsupervised learning is also identified for feature removal, whereas supervised learning is appropriate for analytical representation by constructing several interactions involving patient individuality (input) and result of concern (output). In recent times, semisupervised learning has been projected as a hybrid involving supervised learning and unsupervised learning, which is appropriate for circumstances wherever the effect is omitted for definite issues.

There are two major unsupervised learning techniques available such as (i) principal component analysis (PCA) technique and (ii) clustering technique. Principal component analysis is basically for element reduction, mainly while the characteristic is documented in a huge number of elements, such as the number of genes in a genome-mixt connection revise. Principal component analyses (PCA) project the data on a small number of principal component (PC) guidelines, without trailing in excess of information regarding the issues. Occasionally, PCA is used to decrease the element of the data, after which clustering technique is used to fraction the issues. All these fraction issues with related characteristics are gathered together, without applying any result information. This algorithm's result output helps the cluster tags for the patients throughout maximizing as well as minimizing the parallel of the patients and also involving the clusters. These accepted clustering algorithms contain (i) Gaussian mixture clustering, (ii) K-means clustering, and (iii) hierarchical clustering. Alternatively, supervised learning reflects on the topics' outcomes in cooperation with their characteristics and goes via a definite training procedure to find out the finest outputs connected through the inputs, which are nearby the standard outcomes. Generally, the formulations of output contrast through the concern outcomes. Such that, the outcome can be the possibility of receiving an exact clinical result, the projected value of a disease stage or the projected endurance time. Evaluated by unsupervised learning and supervised learning, which offers extra clinically applicable results; therefore Artificial Intelligence (AI) relevance in healthcare system most regularly apply supervised learning. Unsupervised learning may be applied as a component of the preprocessing stage to or find out subgroups or decrease dimensionality, which consecutively makes summarizing supervised learning stage more capable. Appropriate methods contain logistic regression, linear regression, decision tree, naïve Bayes, random forest, discriminate analysis, nearest neighbor, neural network, and support vector machine (SVM). Neural network and SVM are the most accepted supervised learning methods in healthcare applications [5]. The mechanisms of neural networks and support vector machine (SVM) techniques process together with relevant examples in the cardiovascular disease, neurological disease, and cancer.

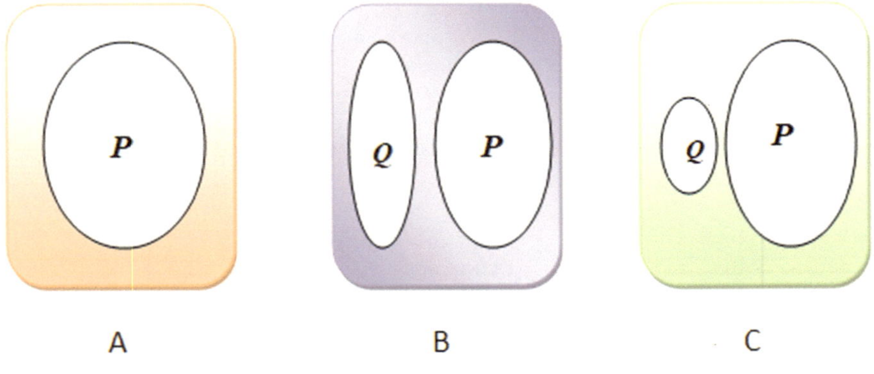

Figure 2.
Representation of (A) unsupervised learning, (B) supervised learning, and (C) semisupervised learning.

2.2 Neural network

Neural network is basically known as the expansion of linear regression for confining the difficult nonlinear relationships dividing the input parameters and outcome data. In this neural network, the relations involving the input parameters and the outcome are represented throughout the multiple unknown layer grouping of preindividual functional. The aim is to calculate approximately the weights via input data and also the outcome data so that the average error involving the outcome and their calculation is reduced. Here, this technique is described via following some examples. Neural network was used in stroke diagnosis [6], where the input parameters were given as $Xi_1, \ldots, X_{ip}$ and $p = 16$ stroke-related symptoms, together with acute confusion, problem of vision and mobility, paresthesia of the leg or arm, etc. Y_i represents the binary outcome, where $Y_i = 1/0$ represents that the ith patient has or does not have stroke. The output factor of importance is the possibilities of stroke (a_i), which represents the equation given below:

$$a_i = h\left\{\sum_{K=1}^{D} w2l\, fk\left(\sum_{l=1}^{p} w1l\, X_{il} + w_{10}\right) + w_{20}\right\} \tag{1}$$

In this equation, w_{10} and w_{20} are not equal to zero, where $X_{ij}, fk = 0; fk$s and h are prespecified functions, which indicate that the weighted grouping influences the disease threat as a whole. **Figure 3** represents the neural network system.

The instruction's aim is to find out the weight of w_{ij}, which can minimize the calculation in accuracy given by $\Sigma_{i=1}^{n}(Y_i - a_i)^2$. The minimization can be done via standard optimization algorithms, for instance, local quadratic estimate or gradient decline optimization, which are integrated in both R and MATLAB software. The latest data were issued from the similar population and the results of w_{ij} are also applied to calculate the outcomes rooted in their particular characters [7]. This is the same as methods have been applied to identify cancer treatment [8], where the input efforts and outcomes are the principal components (PC) predictable from 6567 genes and the tumor groups. A neural network was applied to identify breast cancer, where the inputs represent the surface information from mammographic images and where the outcomes are tumor indicators [9]. Another problematical neural network model was analyzed to identify Parkinson's disease derived where the input parameters are motor and nonmotor indications and neuroimages [10].

2.3 The support vector machine (SVM)

The supporting vector machine is mostly applied for categorizing the topics into two different clusters, where the result Y_i, $Y_i = -1$ or 1 indicates whether the ith patient is in set 1 or 2 correspondingly. This procedure can be completed for circumstances with more than 2 sets. The fundamental hypothesis is that the subject matters can be divided into two different groups via a decision boundary distinct on the characteristics Xij, which can be represented as:

$$a_i = \sum_{j=1}^{p} w_j X_{ij} + b \tag{2}$$

where w_j represents the weight put on the jth characteristic to mark edits' comparative implication on moving the outcome between the others. If $a_i > 0$, the ith patient is categorized to group 1, that is, $Y_i = -1$; and if $a_i < 0$, the patient is categorized to group 2, that is, $Y_i = 1$. Furthermore, assuming that the new patients come from the same population, the resulting W_j can be applied to classify these new patients based on their traits. An important property of SVM is that the determination of the model parameters is a convex optimization problem so the solution

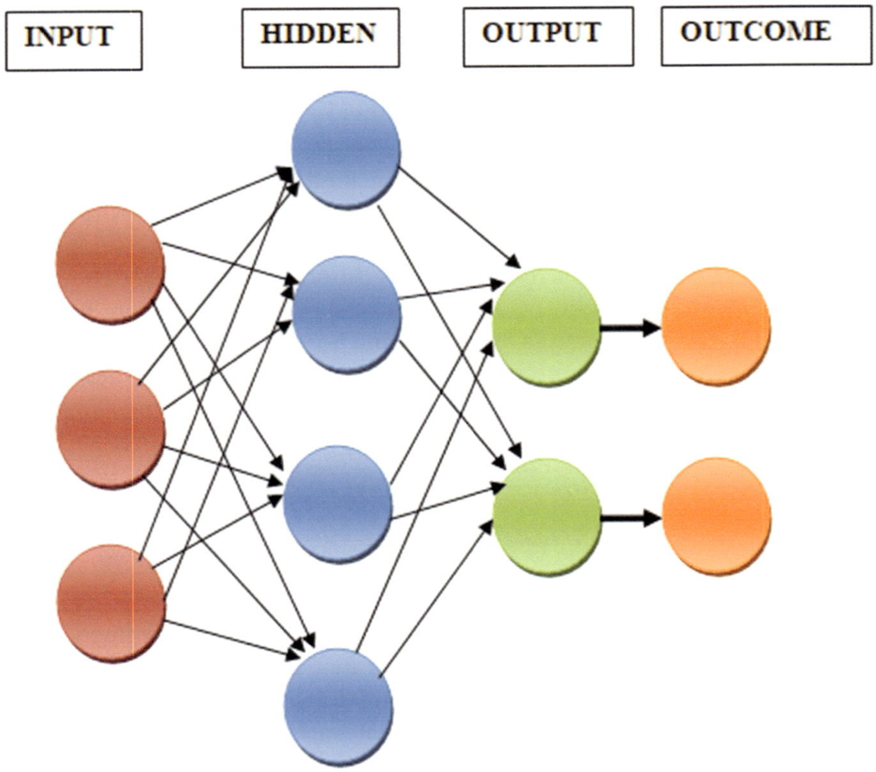

Figure 3.
Neural network diagram.

is always global optimum. Additionally, many obtainable rounded optimization technique applications are readily available for the SVM performance. SVM has been widely applied in healthcare research. For example, SVM was used to recognize imaging biomarkers of psychiatric and neurological disease [11]. SVM was also applied in cancer diagnosis [12]. SVM and other statistical methods can also be used to reach early detection of Alzheimer's syndrome [13]. SVM was applied to analyze the power of an offline human and device interface, which can control the upper-limb prostheses [14].

2.4 Deep learning method

Deep learning method is a contemporary expansion of the traditional neural network method. **Figure 4** represents deep learning like a neural network with multicovers.

Rapid growth of current computing allowed deep learning for constructing the neural networks along with huge amount of covers, which is impossible for traditional neural networks. Basically, this technique helps to investigate many critical nonlinear models in the information. One more cause for the recent acceptance of deep learning techniques is owing to the enhancement of the critical and volume of data [15]. Dissimilar to the traditional neural network, this process generally applies more hidden levels in order that the algorithms can handle critical data with different structures [5]. In the healthcare applications, the generally applied deep learning algorithms consist of recurrent neural network, convolution neural network technique, deep neural network, and deep belief network. Convolution neural network is the most accepted one in 2016. The convolution neural network is extended to analyzing the ineptitude of the traditional machine learning algorithms when conducting high dimensional data, that is, data with a huge number of characteristics. Conventionally, the machine learning algorithms are considered to examine data when the number of characteristics is little. The image data are physically high dimensional because each image generally includes thousands of pixels as characteristics. One explanation is to present dimension decrease: primarily preselect an object of pixels as elements and then complete the machine learning algorithms on the ensuing lower dimensional traits. However, heuristic feature selection events may drop the information in the images. Unsupervised learning methods such as clustering or PCA can be applied for data-determined dimension decrease. The convolution neural network was first projected the high-dimensional image investigation [16], where the inputs for convolution neural network are the accurately regulated pixel values on the images. The convolution neural network then transmitted the pixel values in the image throughout weighting in the difficulty layers and variety in the subsampling layers instead. The ultimate output is a recursive purpose of the weighted input values. The weights are skilled to reduce the average error involving the predictions and the outcomes. The performance of convolution neural network has been incorporated in trendy software packages such as Caffe from Berkeley AI Research [17] and Tensor Flow from Google [18]. Recently, the convolution neural network has been effectively executed in the healthcare area to help disease identification. It is used to identify the congenital cataract disease throughout learning the ocular images [19], though it has over 90% accuracy on identification and treatment implication. Convolution neural network was performed to identify skin cancer from clinical images [20]. Convolution neural network is applied to identify referable diabetic retinopathy via the retinal fundus photographs [21]. The specificity and sensitivity of the algorithm are both over 90%, which expressed the usefulness of using the method in the analysis of diabetes. It is importance to declare that in all this type of applications, the presentation of the convolution neural network is competitive beside an experienced physician in the truthfulness for categorizes both usual and disease stages.

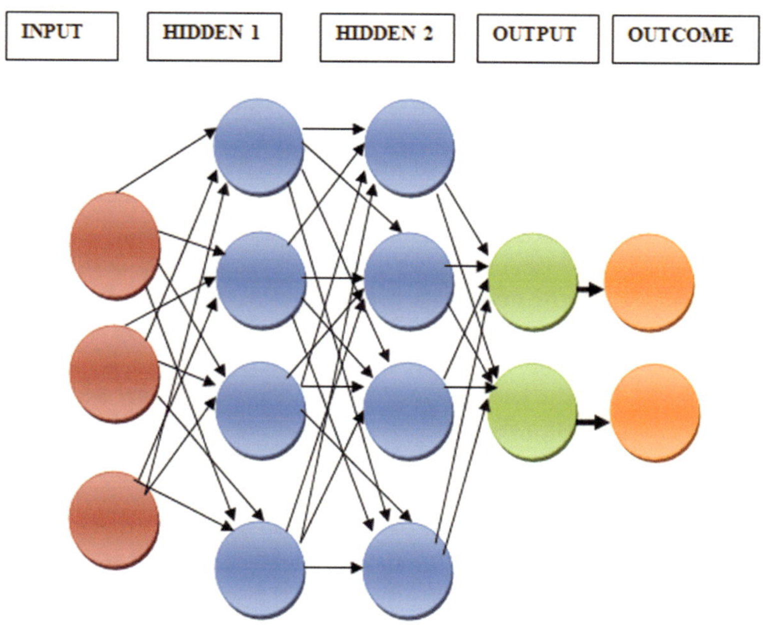

Figure 4.
Multilayer neural network.

2.5 Natural language processing

Genetic data and EP plus image are all machine-comprehensible, that is why the machine learning (ML) algorithms can be straightly presented after quality control processes or appropriate preprocessing. Though huge extents of medical data are like descriptive content, like a substantial examination, operative notes, and an experimental laboratory reports and release abstracts, these are formless and inconceivable for computer programming. Below this background, natural language processing (NLP) targets removing helpful data from the descriptive text to support the medical conclusion making [3]. A natural language processing (NLP) pipeline includes two main components: (i) classification and (ii) text processing. During text processing, the natural language processing (NLP) recognizes a sequence of disease-appropriate keywords at clinical remarks related to the past records [22]. After that, keyword subsets are preferred during analyzing their achievements in the arrangement in the normal abnormal cases. The authorized keywords then enter and enhance the controlled information to support medical choice making. The natural language processing pipelines have been developed to help the medical choice making on attentive treatment preparations and monitoring critical effects. For instance, it was showed that establishment of natural language processing, for analyzing the chest X-ray reports would help the antibiotic assistant system to aware physicians for the probable necessitate for anti-infective therapy [23]. Natural language processing was used to mechanically monitor laboratory-based difficult effects. Moreover, the natural language processing pipelines can also assist with disease analysis [24]. A recognized of 14 cerebral aneurysm disease-associated changeable during executing natural language processing (NLP), based on the clinical remarks [25]. Resulting variables are effectively applied for categorizing the common patients and the patients with cerebral problems, with 86% to 95% accuracy rates on the validation and training trials correspondingly. A natural language processing was implemented to extort the peripheral arterial disease-allied keywords from description clinical remarks. The keywords are then applied to categorize the common patients and the patients who have peripheral arterial disease, which reaches over 90% accurate [22].

3. Artificial intelligence (AI) applications in healthcare system

In spite of few limitations, artificial intelligence (AI) are applied in healthcare system. Researchers mainly focus on the region of major three diseases: cardiovascular disease, nervous system disease, and life-threatening cancer also. In cardiology, [26] explained the prospective uses of the AI system for making a diagnosis of the cardiac diseases with the help of cardiac images. Cardiac stroke is a natural and commonly stirring disease that has an effect on more than 500 million people all around the world. It is the most leading cause of death in world. It has also high medical expenses across the world nearly about US$ 689 billion, which causes serious trouble to patient families [27, 28]. For that reason, research on anticipation and medical treatment for stroke has a great impact. Recently, artificial intelligence (AI) processes have been used in additional and supplementary stroke-connected studies. In stroke-concerned cases, AI procedures help in the three main areas: before time for disease calculation and analysis, healing, and in addition to conclusion forecast and diagnosis assessment. About 85% of the time, stroke is caused by cerebral infarction, that is, thrombus in the vessel. For require of finding pre stroke indication, only some patients could obtain appropriate treatment. A movement-detecting device was developed for predicting early stroke [29]. For model structure resolution, two machine learning algorithms like PCA and genetic fuzzy finite state machine are mainly used. The revealing method is attached with a patient human action detection phase and the starting of the stroke detection phase. Ideally, the typical model is remarkably different from the patient movement, and an attentive model that can detect stroke can stimulate and assess medical action and make it immediately feasible. Correspondingly, a device that is wearable was proposed for gathering data for regular and pathological steps for calculation of stroke [30]. The data can be removed and copied by SVM and unseen Markov models, and this algorithm could suitably organize 91% of information to the exact group. For some identification of the stroke, neuro-imaging processes like CT scan and MRI are also essential for disease estimation. Several studies have attempted to concern machine learning techniques to neuro-imaging data to support with stroke analysis. SVM was used in resting-state functional MRI data, where endophenotypes of motor disability behind stroke were classified and recognized [31]. This algorithm can precisely distinguish patients with a precision of 87.6%. T1-weighted MRI, [32] helps to rearrange the stroke injury. This effect is similar for human-proficient physical injury explanation. Kamnitsas et al. [33] attempted 3D CNN aimed at injury fragmentation in multisculpt brain MRI. It likewise used fully associated provisional casual field representation for ultimate postprocessing of the CNN's soft segmentation plots. With the help of Gaussian process regression method, stroke anatomical MRI images were analyzed,and also establish the vortex pattern performed well than injury load/area like the expecting elements [34]. Machine learning (ML) techniques are also useful to examine stroke patients with CT scans. A free-floating intraluminal thrombus can be created like injury post stroke, and this is complicated to discriminate by carotid sign in CT imaging. Three machine learning (ML) algorithms were used to categorize two quantitative types: shape analysis with linear classification analysis, SVM, and artificial neural network [35]. Machine learning is also used in expecting and evaluating the presentation for stroke cure. In a critical emergency phase determination, the result of intravenous thrombolysis (tPA) has a sturdy link for the diagnosis per durance rate. With CT scan, SVM can be used for expecting whether the patients by thrombolysis (tPA) cure can build up suggestive intracranial hemorrhage [36]. In SVM, complete brain images were used as input, which acted healthier than traditional radiology-based procedures. For improving the medical result making procedure of thrombolysis (tPA) healing, a stroke treatment model was proposed for investigating perform guiding principle, clinical trials and meta-analysis with Bayesian principle network [37]. The model consisted of 56 different types of variables and 3 decisions aimed at investigating the process for analysis, cure, and effective calculation. An interaction tree was used, where the subgroup investigated suitable thrombolysis (tPA) dosage as per patient individuality, taking into consideration the healing efficacy and the possibility of bleeding [38]. Several issues can influence stroke diagnosis and syndrome mortality. Evaluating with traditional methods, machine learning techniques have returns in progressing calculation activity. To enhance and maintain the medical assessment making procedure, a model was proposed for expecting a three-month healing outcome by examining the physiological considerations for the duration of 48 hours following stroke with logistic degeneration [39]. A database was observed with 107 patient's medical information through acute anterior stroke and also posterior stroke via intra-arterial therapy [18]. Here, the data were examined through SVM and artificial neural network and achieved calculation accurateness of more than 70%. Machine learning procedures was used to recognize the control effect in brain arterio-venous abnormality satisfied with endo-vascular embolization. Though typical degeneration analysis representation could only reach a 43%

precision rate, this technique's exertion is much enhanced with 97.5% exactness. An optimal algorithm was analyzed to calculate 30 days mortality test and gained additional exact calculation than surviving techniques [40]. Likewise, SVM was used to calculate the stroke mortality via discharge. Additionally, the application of the synthetic alternative oversampling procedure was proposed to decrease the stroke effect calculation prejudice reasoned among class inequality between several datasets. Brain images were examined for calculating the effect of stroke cure. CT scan data were examined through machine learning procedure for estimating the cerebral edema through hemispheric infraction [41]. A random forest was constructed to involuntarily recognize the cerebrospinal fluid (CSF) and examined the changes in the CT scan, and this is more precise and capable compared to the traditional procedures. Functional connectivity was extracted from magnetic resonance imaging (MRI) and practical magnetic resonance imaging (MRI) data, and ridge degeneration and multitasking intellect were also applied for cognitive deficit calculation following stroke [42]. A relationship was examined, which involved injuries extorted from magnetic resonance imaging (MRI) and the cure effect through Gaussian method regression technique [43]. The model was used to calculate the difficulty of cognitive damages during stroke and the way of retrieval in due course. In Arterys Cardio DL process, where artificial intelligence (AI) is help to make available programmed and also changeable ventricle segmentations related on traditional MRI of cardiac images [44]. In nervous system disease, an artificial intelligence (AI) method was developed [45] for repairing the regulation of body movement in quadriplegia patients. Farina et al. experienced the control of the offline man–machine edge, which applies the release timings for the spinal motor neurons for controlling the prosthesis of the upper limb. IBM Watson for the oncology diagnosis can be a consistent AI for cancer diagnosis from start to the end, which was explained by Somashekhar et al. [46] by a double-blinded validation study. A clinical image was examined for recognizing skin cancer subtypes [20]. The applications of these three types' diseases are not absolutely unpredicted. These three diseases are principal death causes; for that reason, analyzing the stages of the disease before time is vital to avoid worsening of the patients' health condition. Moreover, quick diagnoses can prospectively reach throughout recovering the analysis measures on electrophysiological (EP) or electronic medical record (EMR), imaging and genetic, and this is the major power of the artificial intelligence (AI) technique. Moreover, apart from the three main diseases, artificial intelligence (AI) system has been used in another disease too: to examine the ocular image data for diagnosing inherited cataract diseases [19]. A referable diabetic retinopathy was detected by the retinal fundus photographs [21].

4. Application of artificial intelligence in modern medicine

Artificial intelligence in modern medicine and medial area has been a mostly upcoming hot topic in current years. Although there is wisdom of excessive prospective in the use of artificial intelligence in modern medicine, there are also worries about the defeat of the 'human touch' in such an important and person-motivated work. Artificial intelligence in modern medicine denotes to the practice of artificial intelligence tools and programmed procedures in the identification and cure of patients who need care. At the same time as analysis and cure may appear like modest phases, there are numerous other circumstantial procedures that come to pass in demand for a patient designate properly taken to attention, such as:

i. Collecting information data from patient discussions and checks

ii. Treating and examining outcomes of result

iii. Applying several causes of information data to derive an exact identification

iv. Defining an applicable cure technique

v. Arranging and controlling the selected cure technique

vi. Patient observing

vii. Rehabilitation, continuation arrangements

Disagreement for enlarged use of artificial intelligence in modern medicine is that reasonably a various of the beyond could be programmed—computerization often means jobs are finished more swiftly, and it also help to frees up the time of a medical expert's when they could be acting other responsibilities, which cannot be computerized, and hence are appreciated as a more cherished practice of human wealth. For instance, technology application has improved in all regions of daily life. Now, there are unbelievable volumes of tools and robotics in association with modern medicine; all medical information is digitized, online appointments can be arranged, and with the help of different healthcare apps in smartphone, it can be easy to find out nearest medical clinics or any health centers. Artificial intelligence is already being used in healthcare modern medicine nowadays. As a medical assessment support system, DXplain [47] is an artificial intelligence system that can help to perform on a set of medical outcomes like symptoms, marks, laboratory files, etc. to make a hierarchical list of identification that can describe the medical indices. Germwatcher [48] is another artificial intelligent system that is considered to notice, and examine taints in needy patients. In medical robotic surgical technology, the "da Vinci robotic surgical system" [49] with defined movement, robotic arms, and magnetized visualization permits surgeons to perform surgery that is not possible through an exclusively manual method. The probable for enlarged artificial intelligence practice in modern medicine is not objective in a decrease of physical jobs and reducing doctor's time, growing proficiency and output-it also offers the prospect for healthcare system to change to further accuracy of modern medicine.

5. Alginate and AI in biomedical fields

Smart biomedical and medical packaging with the application of polymers is a generally and rapidly growing area of interest for academia and industries. Among a variety of polymers such as alginate, many uses have been created such as in biomedical field, medicine, packaging, and food sector [50]. For example, in modern drug delivery systems, a mesh completed of nanofibers created by the electrospinning process is highly desired. Electro-spinning for biomedicine is based on the application of natural substances and biopolymers, along with the mixture of drugs such as sulfisoxazole, naproxen, and essential oils with antibacterial properties such as eugenol and tocopherol. In recent times, there has been an enormous thrust in the usage of biopolymers for a number of applications, especially in the biomedical and also in pharmaceutical areas [51, 52]. The functional effectiveness of the biopolymer molecules depends on the physicochemical properties, structural features, and composition [53]. It is feasible to rationally design the structure and composition of the biopolymer to gain suitable useful features [54]. The internal structure of the polymer molecule determines many functional characteristics, for example permeability, integrity, and chargeability [55]. The strength of the biopolymer particles and their summative capability is influenced by the electrical characteristics. Molecules of biopolymers and their electrical properties influence the contact with other molecules present in the neighboring environment. Alginate is one of the most popular natural biopolymers and intensely studied [56, 57]. It is an anionic biopolymer consisting of units of guluronic acid and mannuronic acid in uneven blocks [58]. Guluronic acid and mannuronic acid are linked by glycosidic linkages [59, 60], whereas the guluronic acid forms α bonds ($1 \rightarrow 4$) and β ($1 \rightarrow 4$) bonds with mannuronic acid [61]. The stiffness of molecular chains is ensured by the rigid and bent conformations of guluronic acid [62]. Hecth et al. have recently discussed their study on the characterization of calcium alginate and sodium alginate with particular importance on their structure [63]. Different applications and properties of alginate have also been examined. Alginate characteristics used biomedical especially in biomedicine can be formed by adjusting the accessibility of their hydroxyl and carboxyl groups [64]. It influences the characteristics of alginates, such as hydrophobicity, solubility, and their biological activity [65]. Alginate hydrogels were formed by cross-linking polymer chains [66]. The chemical properties of alginate hydrogels were found to depend on the cross-linking density of the chain [67]. The cellular viability of MG-63 osteosarcoma cells was improved by blending alginate bioink solution with N-acetyl cysteine (NAC) [68]. One of the techniques used in the design of alginate hydrogels is intermolecular cross-linking, wherein only the alginate guluronan groups react with the divalent cation, most frequently the calcium used to gel the alginate [69].

6. Conclusions

Artificial intelligence (AI) in healthcare offered a variety of healthcare information results that artificial intelligence (AI) has examined and reviewed the most important types of diseases that artificial intelligence (AI) has arranged. Machine learning (ML) and natural language processing are two major groups of artificial intelligence (AI) devices. For machine learning (ML) process, two most accepted traditional methods are available, that is, neural network and SVM. A typical artificial intelligence (AI) system must have the machine learning (ML) component that can help for conducting the structured data such as EP data, images, and genetic data and another natural language processing (NLP) module for the deduction of unstructured works. The complicated algorithm requires to be taught during the healthcare results previous to the system which can support the physicians for the disease analysis and plans which should be required for treatment. This technique focuses on how computer-oriented assessment methods, within the same roof as artificial intelligence (AI), can help in improving health and clinical area. Even though sophisticated information and machine learning present the base for artificial intelligence (AI), at present, there are revolutionary progresses happening in the subfield of neural networks. This has produced remarkable enthusiasm in several fields of healthcare science, as well as drug analysis and public health. Deep neural networks can execute as well as the most excellent human clinicians in definite diagnostic responsibilities. Additionally, artificial intelligence (AI) tools are already emerging in health-based apps, which can be engaged in handheld, network machines such as smart mobile phones. The major obstructions to be defeated in building health and healthcare data information are the space between digital data and human cognition. Data information regarding an entity patient is mostly gained in forms designed to be available to healthcare personnel. Typical data may consist of MRI or X-ray or ultrasound pictures of the patient, visual records of lung or heart function differing with time, or verbal similes of the patient as seen by the medical personnel. Alternatively, when data are accumulated in data information process and applied, in health research or to expand treatment procedures, it is regularly concentrated to statistical information that is mainly digital. The transfer of analog input into digital output is an oppressive task and may result in a defeat of important information, which would have been cooperative to the consumer.

Author details

Sudipto Datta[1*], Ranjit Barua[1] and Jonali Das[2]

1 Centre for Healthcare Science and Technology, Indian Institute of Engineering Science and Technology, Shibpur, Howrah, West Bengal, India

2 Department of Chemistry, Calcutta University, Uttarpara, Hooghly, West Bengal, India

*Address all correspondence to: dattadip440v@gmail.com

References

[1] James G, Witten D, Hastie T, et al. An Introduction to Statistical Learning with Applications in R. 1st ed. Springer; 2013

[2] Darcy AM, Louie AK, Roberts LW. Machine learning and the profession of medicine. JAMA. 2016;**315**:551-552

[3] Christopher DM, Hinrich S. Foundations of Statistical Natural Language Processing. Cambridge, London, England: The MIT Press; 1999

[4] Murff HJ, FitzHenry F, Matheny ME, et al. Automated identification of postoperative complications within an electronic medical record using natural language processing. JAMA. 2011;**306**:848-855

[5] Good fellow I, Bengio Y, Courville A. Deep Learning. 1st ed. Cambridge, London, England: The MIT Press; 2016

[6] Mirtskhulava L, Wong J, Al-Majeed S, Pearce G, et al., editors. Artificial neural network model in stroke diagnosis. In: 2015 17th UKSim-AMSS International Conference on Modelling and Simulation (UKSim). IEEE; 2015

[7] Bishop CM, editor. Pattern Recognition and Machine Learning (Information Science and Statistics); 2007

[8] Khan J, Wei JS, Ringnér M, et al. Classification and diagnostic prediction of cancers using gene expression profiling and artificial neural networks. Nature Medicine. 2001;7:673-679

[9] Dheeba J, Albert Singh N, Tamil Selvi S. Computer-aided detection of breast cancer on mammograms: A swarm intelligence optimized wavelet neural network approach. Journal of Biomedical Informatics. 2014;**49**:45-52

[10] Hirschauer TJ, Adeli H, Buford JA. Computer-aided diagnosis of Parkinson's disease using enhanced probabilistic neural network. Journal of Medical Systems. 2015;**39**:179

[11] Orrù G, Pettersson-Yeo W, Marquand AF, et al. Using support vector machine to identify imaging biomarkers of neurological and psychiatric disease: A critical review. Neuroscience & Biobehavioral Reviews. 2012;**36**:1140-1152

[12] Sweilam NH, Tharwat AA, Abdel Moniem NK, Moniem NKA. Supportvector machine for diagnosis cancer disease: A comparative study. Egyptian Informatics Journal. 2010;**11**:81-92

[13] Khedher L, Ramírez J, Górriz JM, et al. Early diagnosis of Alzheimer's disease based on partial least squares, principal component analysis and support vector machine using segmented MRI images. Neurocomputing. 2015;**151**:139-150

[14] Farina D, Vujaklija I, Sartori M, et al. Man/machine interface based on the discharge timings of spinal motor neurons after targeted musclere innervation. Nature Biomedical Engineering. 2017;**1**:0025

[15] Ravi D, Wong C, Deligianni F, et al. Deep learning for health informatics. IEEE Journal of Biomedical and Health Informatics. 2017;**21**:4-21

[16] Lecun Y, Bottou L, Bengio Y, et al. Gradient-based learning applied to document recognition. Proceedings of the IEEE (Inst Electr Electron Eng). 1998;**86**:2278-2324

[17] Research BA. Caffe. 2017. Available from: http://caffe.berkeleyvision.org/ [Accessed: 1 June 2017]

[18] Abadi M, Agarwal A, Barham P, et al; Tensor Flow: Large-Scale Machine Learning on Heterogeneous Distributed Systems; 2016

[19] Long E, Lin H, Liu Z, et al. An Artificial Intelligence Platform for the Multihospital Collaborative Management of Congenital Cataracts; 2017

[20] Esteva A, Kuprel B, Novoa RA, et al. Dermatologist-level classification of skin cancer with deep neural networks. Nature. 2017;**542**:115-118

[21] Gulshan V, Peng L, Coram M, et al. Development and validation of deep learning algorithm for detection of diabetic retinopathy in retinal fundus photographs. JAMA. 2016;**316**:2402-2410

[22] Afzal N, Sohn S, Abram S, et al. Mining peripheral arterial disease cases from narrative clinical notes using natural language processing. Journal of Vascular Surgery. 2017;**65**:1753-1761

[23] Fiszman M, Chapman WW, Aronsky D, et al. Automatic detectionof acute bacterial pneumonia from chest X-ray reports. Journal of the American Medical Informatics Association. 2000;7:593-604

[24] Miller TP, Li Y, Getz KD, et al. Using electronic medical record data toreport laboratory adverse events. British Journal of Haematology. 2017;**177**:283-286

[25] Castro VM, Dligach D, Finan S, et al. Large-scale identification of patients with cerebral aneurysms using natural language processing. Neurology. 2017;**88**:164-168

[26] Dilsizian SE, Siegel EL. Artificial intelligence in medicine and cardiac imaging: Harnessing big data and advanced computing to provide personalized medical diagnosis and treatment. Current Cardiology Reports. 2014;**16**:441

[27] Saenger AK, Christenson RH. Stroke biomarkers: Progress and challenges for diagnosis, prognosis, differentiation, and treatment. Clinical Chemistry. 2010;**56**:21-33

[28] Heeley E, Anderson CS, Huang Y, et al. Role of health insurance inverting economic hardship in families after acute stroke in China. Stroke. 2009;**40**:2149-2156

[29] Villar JR, González S, Sedano J, et al. Improving human activity recognition and its application in early stroke diagnosis. International Journal of Neural Systems. 2015;**25**:1450036

[30] Mannini A, Trojaniello D, Cereatti A, et al. A machine learning framework for gait classification using inertial sensors: Application to elderly, post-stroke and Huntington's disease patients. Sensors. 2016;**16**:134

[31] Rehme AK, Volz LJ, Feis DL, et al. Identifying neuroimaging markers of motor disability in acute stroke by machine learning techniques. Cerebral Cortex. 2015;**25**:3046-3056

[32] Griffis JC, Allendorfer JB, Szaflarski JP. Voxel-based Gaussian naïve Bayes classification of ischemic stroke lesions in individual T1-weighted MRI scans. Journal of Neuroscience Methods. 2016;**257**:97-108

[33] Kamnitsas K, Ledig C, Newcombe VF, et al. Efficient multi-scale3D CNN with fully connected CRF for accurate brain lesion segmentation. Medical Image Analysis. 2017;**36**:61-78

[34] Rondina JM, Filippone M, Girolami M, et al. Decoding post-stroke motor function from structural brain imaging. NeuroImage: Clinical. 2016;**12**:372-380

[35] Thornhill RE, Lum C, Jaberi A, et al. Can shape analysis differentiate free-floating internal carotid artery Thrombus from atherosclerotic plaque in patients evaluated with CTA? For stroke or transient ischemic attack? Academic Radiology. 2014;**21**:345-354

[36] Bentley P, Ganesalingam J, Carlton Jones AL, et al. Prediction of stroke thrombolysis outcome using CT brain machine learning. NeuroImage: Clinical. 2014;**4**:635-640

[37] Love A, Arnold CW, El-Saden S, et al. Unifying acute stroke treatment guidelines for a bayesian belief network. Studies in Health Technology and Informatics. 2013;**192**:1012

[38] Ye H, Shen H, Dong Y, et al. Using Evidence-Based Medicine through Advanced Data Analytics to Work toward a National Standard for Hospital-Based Acute Ischemic Stroke Treatment. Mainland China; 2017

[39] Zhang Q, Xie Y, Ye P, et al. Acute ischaemic stroke prediction from physiological time series patterns. The Australasian Medical Journal. 2013;**6**:280-286

[40] Birkner MD, Kalantri S, Solao V, et al. Creating diagnostic scores using data-adaptive regression: An application to prediction of 30-day mortality among stroke victims in a rural hospital in India. Therapeutics and Clinical Risk Management. 2007;**3**:475-484

[41] Chen Y, Dhar R, Heitsch L, et al. Automated quantification of cerebral edema following hemispheric infarction: Application of a machine learning algorithm to evaluate CSF shifts on serial head CTs. NeuroImage: Clinical. 2016;**12**:673-680

[42] Siegel JS, Ramsey LE, Snyder AZ, et al. Disruptions of network connectivity predict impairment in multiple behavioral domains after stroke. Proceedings of the National Academy of Sciences of the United States of America. 2016;**113**:E4367-E4376

[43] Hope TM, Seghier ML, Leff AP, et al. Predicting outcome and recovery after stroke with lesions extracted from MRI images. NeuroImage: Clinical. 2013;**2**:424-433

[44] Marr B. First FDA Approval for Clinical Cloud-Based Deep Learning in Healthcare; 2017

[45] Bouton CE, Shaikhouni A, Annetta NV, et al. Restoring cortical control of functional movement in a human with quadriplegia. Nature. 2016;**533**:247-250

[46] Somashekhar SP, Kumarc R, Rauthan A. Abstract S6-07: Double blinded validation study to assess performance of IBM artificial intelligence platform, Watson for oncology in comparison with manipal multidisciplinary tumourboard? First study of 638 breast cancer cases. Cancer Research. 2017;**77**(4 Suppl):S6-S7

[47] Barnett GO, Cimino JJ, Hupp JA, Hoffer EP. DXplain. An evolving diagnostic decision-support system. The Journal of the American Medical Association. 1987;**258**(1):67-74

[48] Khan MG, Steib SA, Dunagan WC, Fraser VJ. Monitoring expert system performance using continuous user feedback. Journal of the American Medical Informatics Association. 1996;**3**:216-223

[49] Rao R, Nayyar R, Panda S, Hemal AK. Surgical techniques: Robotic bladder diverticulectomy with the da Vinci-S surgical system. Journal of Robotic Surgery. 2007;**1**:217-220

[50] Barua R, Datta S, Datta P, RoyChowdhury A. Scaffold and Tissue

Engineering Applications by 3D Bio-Printing Process: A New Approach. IgI Global; 2019. pp. 78-99

[51] Fernando IPS, Kim D, Nah J-W, Jeon Y-J. Advances in functionalizing fucoidans and alginates (bio) polymers by structural modifications: A review. Chemical Engineering Journal. 2019;**355**:33-48

[52] Bayer IS. Thermomechanical properties of polylactic acid-graphene composites: A state-of-the-art review for biomedical applications. Materials. 2017;**10**:748

[53] Madhumitha G, Fowsiya J, Roopan SM, Thakur VK. Recent advances in starch–clay nanocomposites. International Journal of Polymer Analysis and Characterization. 2018;**23**:331-345

[54] Thakur VK, Singha AS. Rapid synthesis, characterization, and physicochemical analysis of biopolymer-based graft copolymers. International Journal of Polymer Analysis and Characterization. 2011;**16**:153-164

[55] Jones OG, McClements DJ. Functional biopolymer particles: Design, fabrication, and applications. Comprehensive Reviews in Food Science and Food Safety. 2010;**9**:374-397

[56] Reakasame S, Boccaccini AR. Oxidized alginate-based hydrogels for tissue engineering applications: A review. Biomacromolecules. 2018;**19**:3-21

[57] Aguero L, Zaldivar-Silva D, Pena L, Dias ML. Alginate microparticles as oral colon drug delivery device: A review. Carbohydrate Polymers. 2017;**168**:32-43

[58] Draget KI, Taylor C. Chemical, physical and biological properties of alginates and their biomedical implications. Food Hydrocolloids. 2011;**25**:251-256

[59] Zia KM, Zia F, Zuber M, Rehman S, Ahmad MN. Alginate based polyurethanes: A review of recent advances and perspective. International Journal of Biological Macromolecules. 2015;**79**:377-387

[60] Venkatesan J, Bhatnagar I, Manivasagan P, Kang K-H, Kim S-K. Alginate composites for bone tissue engineering: A review. International Journal of Biological Macromolecules. 2015;**72**:269-281

[61] Pawar SN, Edgar KJ. Alginate derivatization: A review of chemistry, properties and applications. Biomaterials. 2012;**33**:3279-3305

[62] De Vos P, Faas MM, Strand B, Calafiore R. Alginate-based microcapsules for immunoisolation of pancreatic islets. Biomaterials. 2006;**27**:5603-5617

[63] Hecht H, Srebnik S. Structural characterization of sodium alginate and calcium alginate. Biomacromolecules. 2016;**17**:2160-2167

[64] Datta S, Barua R, Sarkar R, Barui A, RoyChowdhury A, Datta P. Design and Development of Alginate: Poly-L-Lysine Scaffolds by 3D Bio Printing and Studying their Mechanical , Structural and Cell Viability; 2018a

[65] Datta S, Sarkar R, Vyas V, Bhutoria S, Barui A, RoyChowdhury A, et al. Alginate-Honey Bioinks with Improved Cell Responses for Applications as Bioprinted Tissue Engineered Constructs; 2018b

[66] Bhat SD, Aminabhavi TM. Pervaporation separation using sodium alginate and its modified membranes—A review. Separation and Purification Reviews. 2007;**36**:203-229

[67] Datta S, Das A, Sasmal P, Bhutoria S, Roy Chowdhury A, Datta P. Alginate-poly (amino acid) extrusion printed scaffolds for tissue engineering applications. International Journal of Polymeric Materials and Polymeric Biomaterials. 2018c;**0**(0):1-9

[68] Datta S, Das A, RoyChowdhury A, Datta P. Bioink Formulations to Ameliorate Bioprinting-Induced Loss of Cellular Viability; 2019

[69] El-Sherbiny IM. Enhanced pH-responsive carrier system based on alginate and chemically modified carboxymethyl chitosan for oral delivery of protein drugs: Preparation and in-vitro assessment. Carbohydrate Polymers. 2010;**80**:1125-1136